CHAIR YOGA
FOR SENIORS

A STEP-BY-STEP GUIDE TO BUILDING YOUR CORE STRENGTH, IMPROVING YOUR BALANCE, AND INCREASING YOUR MOBILITY FOR **AN ACTIVE AND EMPOWERED LIFE**

RECLAIM THE JOY OF MOVEMENT

WRITTEN BY RACHEL PAIGE

Dedicated to my parents Ted and Sher, and my grandma Stella for their unwavering love and support. And to the memory of my grandparents Floyd, Lucille, and John.

TABLE OF CONTENTS

DHARMA BUMS UNITE!

Whenever I teach clients one-on-one or lead a class or workshop, people ask, "Where can I find more?" Let's connect! Become a member of my Facebook group Chair Yoga for Beginners and Seniors, where you'll find more than 80k folks dedicated to practicing chair yoga worldwide, receive free weekly video content and updates about my latest projects and activities. Being part of a community can motivate you to pursue your goals and give you a sense of belonging and support.

Follow me on :

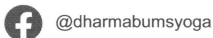 @dharmabumsyoga

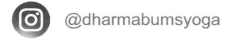 @dharmabumsyoga

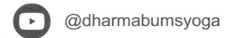 @dharmabumsyoga

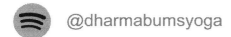 @dharmabumsyoga

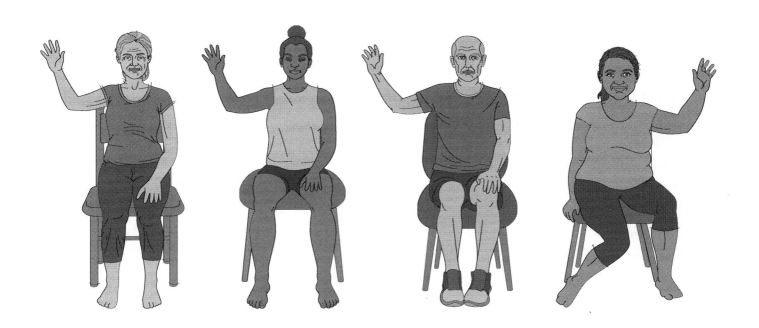

WELCOME!

In this book, I have woven together the lessons I've learned during the past two decades of practicing, studying, and teaching yoga in an easy-to-follow manner. Chair Yoga for Seniors is a comprehensive manual that will instruct you on how to build your core strength, improve your balance, and increase your mobility for an active and empowered life. I am so thrilled that adding a chair for support while doing yoga makes this practice accessible to more people than ever!

Our bodies delight when we take the time to breathe, stretch, and tune them properly. Mentioning the mind-body connection might elicit blank stares or comments that it's only relevant to people who are "woo-woo" or into all that "crazy spiritual stuff," but there is no escaping it. Physical activity doesn't just feel good; it directly correlates to improved emotional well-being and mental health.

Today nearly 27% of adults and seniors do not meet the physical activity levels suggested by the World Health Organization: thirty minutes of moderate exercise, such as brisk walking five days a week, or an hour and fifteen minutes a week of vigorous activities, such as hiking, jogging, or running.

Quite understandably, pain is a significant reason many people don't exercise enough. Whether you're dealing with an illness, injury, surgery, or the consequences of a sedentary lifestyle, many typical exercise routines don't fit the bill or are downright impossible. So, what's the solution?

Chair Yoga for Seniors is your guide to reclaiming the joy of movement. Adding these routines to your weekly exercise routine is a surefire way to help you reach your physical activity goals. It features thirteen accessible yoga routines, including ten and twenty-minute full-body routines, that target the body from head to toe. Each chapter includes a brief description of the anatomical structures of that area, common injuries, and a comprehensive chair yoga workout. You will gain strength, flexibility, and balance for increased longevity.

Physical activity is the foundation of disease prevention and management, including coronary heart disease, hypertension, and type-2 diabetes. It reduces the risk of developing breast and colon cancer, strengthens bones and muscles, enhances brain health, including cognitive function and academic performance, and helps to prevent falls among older adults. In Chapter 5, you'll learn all about the balance system and how to strengthen it to ensure long-term mobility.

Worldwide, levels of anxiety and depression spiked by more than 25% during the Covid pandemic. The unprecedented levels of stress our society faced during this massive upheaval wreaked havoc on the mental health of millions of people, and the long-term consequences of this are yet to be seen.

Today, nearly one in four adults over 18 in the United States has a diagnosable mental health disorder. It's crucial to find outlets that support your well-being. Asking for help when needed is a sign of strength. Sharing your experience with a trusted family member, friend, teacher, mentor, or therapist can help. There are also free and subscription-based online and in-person support groups.

Chair yoga can complement many other therapeutic approaches, including psychoanalysis, behavioral therapy, cognitive therapy, humanistic therapy, integrative or holistic therapy, and medication. It is proven to reduce anxiety and depression in participants. Research your insurance plan and the mental health resources in your area to see what kind of assistance you may be eligible to receive.

In Chapter 3, you will learn more about the importance and role of breath, the most powerful tool to regulate and self-soothe your mind and body. Chair Yoga for Seniors introduces various pranayama (breath control) methods to help you breathe better and increase your lung capacity. It's never too late to tap into the benefits of conscious breathing.

In Chapter 15, you will explore mindfulness, the art of bringing your full awareness to the present with acceptance. Chair Yoga for Seniors will help you shed the layers of protection you've built around your heart and release old patterns of contraction. Meditation nurtures all of the ingredients for a tranquil state of mind: patience, empathy, and compassion.

When you're not healthy and happy, it can be easy to feel your life's purpose is just out of reach. Getting fit for health's sake is not imaginative enough – at least, not for the long term. When you feel at ease in your body, your mental outlook shifts to the positive side. Chair yoga makes it possible to do workouts that invite you to reconnect with your body and start from where you are. You'll find you have the energy to move in the direction of your dreams and to create the life you want to live. You are worth it!

ABOUT ME

My name is **Rachel Paige**, and I'm the founder of Dharma Bums Yoga. One fateful autumn day more than twenty years ago, I stepped through the threshold of my first yoga class. I remember how the instructor taught us tree pose, cueing us to fix our gaze on a tree as we embodied rootedness while seeking balance and reaching for the light. Countless tree poses later, and I am guiding others to slow down and attune themselves to these humble principles that are such a beautiful reflection of life.

Yoga has anchored me through five international moves, fifteen-plus years living abroad, a divorce, and struggles with depression, anxiety, and chronic disease. Whenever I moved to a new country, I attended yoga classes in the local language. I followed along with a watchful eye and picked up new vocabulary as I learned to speak these languages and deepen my yoga practice. I loved that there were spaces far from home where I could reconnect with this ancient practice in a global community of like-minded people.

I am a 200-hour Registered Yoga Teacher (RYT) in Hatha Yoga, completed a 250-hour Ayurveda training, and have studied more than 600 hours of additional coursework in anatomy, physiology, and kinesiology. I am currently studying for a 500-hour certification in circular breathing techniques. I am constantly impressed, though not surprised, by how the ancient yogic teachings consistently prove their physiologic and psychologic benefits in scientific study after scientific study.

Until the Covid-19 pandemic, I taught corporate yoga in Barcelona, Spain. A few months after the start of the lockdown in Spain, I was diagnosed with Meniere's disease. This chronic inner-ear malady impacts balance, and symptoms include hearing loss, tinnitus, inner ear pressure, and vertigo attacks. This strangely named and incurable disease has given me firsthand insight into living with a health condition that severely impacts one's quality of life. It's not an easy reality to cope with or accept, and the adage is too true: "You don't know what you've got till it's gone."

I returned to the United States to find a way forward after my diagnosis. I was drawn back to my family and began caring for my grandparents. It gave me insight into the interventions that made their daily routine more manageable, including optimizing their living space ergonomically and assisting them in rehabilitative exercises when necessary. Caretaking was an intimate experience that showed me the importance of regular exercise and activity for retaining mental clarity, mobility, and independence.

Teaching yoga during that terrifying and uncertain time became an anchor of purpose for me. It was necessary to meet myself and others in a new way, both as a practitioner and a teacher. It quickly became evident that I'd need to modify my teaching style to accommodate my diagnosis. Certain poses became impossible to practice because they could trigger a vertigo attack. In addition, I became mindful of the various health conditions that impacted my older students, including chronic pain, high blood pressure, reduced stamina, and joint replacements. Using the chair during yoga practice was an obvious way to make yoga more accessible.

These experiences were a powerful impetus to deepen my knowledge of the human body. I am fascinated by the structures and systems of the body and strive to share what I know with students in an approachable and easy-to-understand way. This book provides a clear and coherent foundation for you to explore chair yoga at your leisure.

I've helped thousands of students strengthen their mind-body connection, empowering them to connect with the innate joy that occurs when movement, infused by breath and positive intention, releases their limiting beliefs and relieves long-held aches and pains. It's not easy, but the most worthwhile endeavors rarely are. I love my work and students and am honored and excited to share Chair Yoga for Seniors with you. May this book guide you toward greater health, happiness, and fulfillment!

C H A P T E R 1 | ALL ABOUT CHAIR YOGA

Overview

It's time to reclaim the joy of movement! Chair yoga is a practice that will invite you to feel more comfortable with your body and honor its capacities, edges, and innate rhythms. When you connect your breath with movement and presence, a subtle change is set in motion. You may find that instead of treating aches, pains, and anxiety that might creep up during the day as inconveniences, you intuitively remedy them with a slow deep breath and thoughtful stretch instead of sweeping them under the rug. Chair Yoga for Seniors invites you to attend to your needs with kindness and compassion.

Benefits of Chair Yoga

The benefits of chair yoga are multitudinous! Chair yoga can help relieve everyday aches and pains, improve balance, increase strength, boost muscle strength and flexibility, prevent falls, and increase joint range of motion. It helps lower blood pressure, slow the heart rate, and reduce cortisol and adrenaline levels – two hormones associated with higher abdominal fat.

Deep breathing increases blood oxygen levels and enhances internal organ function. Movement and diaphragmatic breathing encourage lymphatic drainage, boosting the immune system.

Meditation can help you manage and reduce anxiety, frustration, and anger. It improves cognitive function, concentration, and problem-solving abilities. It promotes better sleep and boosts happiness levels.

This book provides the tools to begin a comprehensive chair yoga practice that targets the whole body through yoga asana (postures), pranayama (breath exercises), and meditation.

Try Chair Yoga if You:

Want to reclaim the joy of movement – Chair Yoga for Seniors consists of thirteen fun, gentle, and accessible routines that will help you to build core strength, improve your balance and increase your mobility for an active and empowered life.

Don't see yourself as the "type" of person to do yoga – Anyone can do chair yoga. You don't have to be a certain age or have a specific body type, gender, religion, race, or class. It is, as the name suggests, yoga with a chair. The chair is a prop that provides additional support and stability during your yoga routine. It opens the practice to a wide range of individuals keen on exploring a new approach to yoga.

Don't think you're flexible "enough" – Contrary to popular belief, yoga isn't about doing crazy backbends or folding oneself into a pretzel! You don't have to be a former gymnast or dancer to begin. Think of yoga as a lubricant for muscles and joints. Restricted flexibility is all the more reason to get started. Chair yoga will help you stay mobile and independent.

Are recovering from injury, illness, or surgery – Chair yoga makes it possible to stabilize and rest the injured area as you condition the unaffected parts of your body. Injuries and recovery time can be very discouraging, especially when you cannot participate in your favorite activities. Inactivity can snowball into decreased strength, flexibility, and stamina during recuperation. Chair Yoga for Seniors will help motivate you to maintain your capacity in these three key areas.

Have been diagnosed with a chronic or life-threatening illness – A chronic or life-threatening disease diagnosis can feel like a rude loss of autonomy, the arrival of an intrusive and unexpected houseguest you do not wish to host. Breathwork and meditation exercises can be especially beneficial for coping with pain, fear, and the overwhelming loss of control that these experiences can provoke. Chair yoga will support you on your healing journey.

Work regularly in a seated position or have a sedentary lifestyle – Common complaints for those who work all day in a seated position include neck and back pain, muscle tenderness and aches, numb legs, and varicose veins. Additional sedentary lifestyle risks include metabolic syndrome, diabetes, heart disease, and compromised mental health. Chair yoga will teach you helpful stretches, breathing techniques, and meditations to empower you to create positive new habits in your daily routine.

Have limited mobility or a disability – It's possible to adapt chair yoga for people with disabilities, people who use wheelchairs, and those with health conditions that can limit mobility, including arthritis or multiple sclerosis (MS). You can safely and efficiently mobilize your joints and strengthen your muscles during chair yoga without supporting your entire body weight. These exercises can ease everyday movements such as reaching up, folding, bending, and straightening the limbs.

Pull Up a Seat

Chair yoga has the potential to bring the many positive benefits of yoga practice to a wider range of people than ever before. Before beginning any new exercise routine, consult a certified healthcare provider to ensure that chair yoga is the right fit for you. Before your doctor's visit, prepare a list of questions and concerns.

During your practice, remember to pay close attention to your body. Stop if something doesn't feel good or a particular movement causes pain. Pain signals are the body's way of guarding itself. Pushing through it can cause an injury, exacerbate existing injuries, and reinjure old wounds. The chair makes it possible to adjust the yoga poses to benefit your body and protect it from harm.

Mild discomfort may occur when holding a stretch, especially when first starting. Slow deep breaths can help you sustain the depth and duration of your stretch. Respect your body's threshold or time limit for holding a pose. Please don't overdo it!

When you first begin, sustaining specific movements or positions for one or two deep breaths is normal. Regular practice will help you to gain strength and endurance. Training the body to engage in a new activity requires patience and practice.

Chair yoga practice can help you improve your range of motion. The body has nearly 360 joints. That's a lot of points of friction and potential pain. Most people have asymmetrical flexibility and range of motion in their muscles and joints. That means that one side of the body has more or less flexibility and movement than the other, which is normal. Chair yoga allows you to explore your body's boundaries and slowly but surely, increase your natural range of motion. The objective is to meet your body where it is, with acceptance.

If you are aware that you have balance issues or get dizzy quickly, this can indicate an elevated fall risk. Try practicing your routine with a friend, a loved one, or an assistant. In addition, ensure the space you practice in is well-padded and has additional support. A nearby wall can help. Position yourself so that you are stable in your seat, even if the directions recommend that you sit near the edge of the chair. Stability and safety come first.

Feel free to enlist the expertise of an occupational therapist who can provide a home assessment to ensure you can accomplish your daily tasks efficiently. That might mean reorganizing your cupboards and closets for easy access, adding strategic railings in and around your home, booster seats in the bathroom, and incorporating adjustable chairs and beds. Sometimes, simple adjustments can make a world of difference.

Essential Gear and Best Practices

Stability is vital to safe practice. Just as you wouldn't stand on a rickety old chair to grab something from the cupboard, don't entrust that chair to support your precious duff! I highly advise practicing chair yoga on a sturdy wooden chair with a yoga mat rolled out underneath to prevent slippage. Heavy-duty aluminum chairs will also do the trick, but be careful with standing and balance poses as the chair may be less stable and prone to sliding when you lean on it. Simple seated poses and stretches are possible in an office chair, but avoid balance or lunge poses since the wheels and arms on the chair can be dangerous.

Avoid practicing with your feet dangling from the chair, as this can compromise your ability to do the exercises safely. Your feet should touch flat on the floor. If your feet do not touch a solid surface, you can place books or yoga blocks below them. Use cushions or blankets to adjust the seat height if your chair is too low. If you practice in a wheelchair, ensure that you are secure in your seat and use safety precautions, such as locking the brakes, wearing a seat belt if necessary, and doing the routines with assistance.

Additional Gear

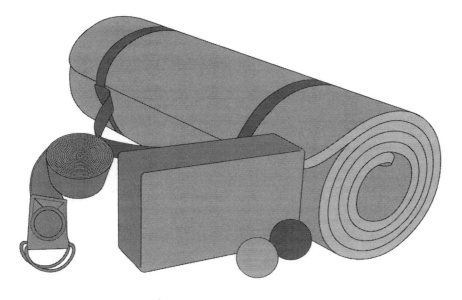

CHAPTER 2 | GETTING STARTED

The use of props during yoga practice is widespread; blankets, bolsters, blocks, straps, foam rollers, and yoga balls are standard. These items can help you modify poses and make practicing more accessible and comfortable. You can substitute these props with everyday household items.

Yoga Mat – A yoga mat will prevent your chair from slipping during exercise. Find one with gripping properties instead of a simple foam mat.

Yoga Balls – Yoga balls are a set of two small balls that you can use in various exercises. You can squeeze them to increase your grip strength, relieve sore feet by rolling them underfoot, and even place one between a sore muscle and a wall to release tension. Tennis balls are excellent substitutes.

Yoga Blocks – Yoga blocks are great props to help modify poses. If, for example, you find it difficult to touch the floor comfortably during an exercise, you can place the block below your hand and use it as support. You can use a thick, hardcover book as an alternative.

Yoga Belt – A yoga belt is a thick nylon band used to stretch and improve the range of motion in both the hips and shoulders. You can also use a belt or a strong scarf.

Music Stand – A music stand can be great when you practice with a book to keep it at eye level as you follow along.

Create a Routine

Set Time Aside – A routine can take up to two weeks to establish, so create a schedule and stick to it. Practicing with friends or small groups can help you stay motivated. Create a distraction-free zone where you can focus on your breath, movement, and peace of mind and learn to tune out the distractions.

Create a Space – You'll want to practice where you can move freely and extend your arms and legs fully. If possible, make this place as inspiring to you as possible. Add elements to it that make you feel good, perhaps a houseplant or a poster with a motivational phrase, or set up a little altar of treasures. Incense or essential oil diffusers help to create a relaxing sensory experience that you link to your chair yoga practice.

Choose Your Music – Listen to something upbeat if you want to feel inspired or something relaxing when you're feeling extra stressed. If you use Spotify, you can find some great playlists on Dharma Bums Yoga; search for my profile. Focus and Concentrate are the ones I listened to as I wrote this book!

Dress Comfortably – Wear comfortable, non-restrictive clothing. Yoga pants and T-shirts are good options. Avoid clothing that is too loose or too tight. No jeans or pants with a tight waistband!

When to Practice – It's best to practice chair yoga with an empty belly. A full stomach can make it hard to take a deep breath, and it may be uncomfortable to do certain poses when your body is busy digesting your food. If you have time in the morning, drink a large glass of water, and if you need some energy, eat a small piece of fruit before practicing. Likewise, you can try to fit in time to practice before dinner or bed, which can be a fantastic way to invite a deep night's rest.

How to Create Your Routine – While going through these yoga routines, you may find specific postures or movements resonate more than others. Choose your favorite exercises from each chapter and combine them to create your own routine. The full-body ten or twenty-minute routines outlined in Chapters 14 and 15 provide good templates for how to do this. If you have a specific area you cannot exercise, continue to condition the body parts you can use.

Incorporate New Healthy Habits

Chair yoga complements many other healthy habits that keep you energized and strong. Once you start practicing chair yoga daily or weekly, you might feel inspired to take additional positive steps to care for yourself. The following are just a few suggestions.

A Healthy Diet – Good nutrition can impact mental and physical health. If you have access to seasonal fresh vegetables and fruits, try incorporating more of them into your diet, and try a new fruit or vegetable once a month. Eat more whole grains, calcium-rich meals, healthy fats, and lean, high-quality protein. Try limiting or cutting out refined sugars and starches. If you have a small patch of land, consider planting a garden to provide your family with fresh produce. If you live in a city, try cultivating fresh herbs on the windowsill to enliven your home cooking.

Hydration – Drink more water! Optimally you want to drink a half gallon of water a day. That's two liters or eight 8-oz glasses daily. Get into the habit of drinking a big glass of water first thing in the morning. If you aren't crazy about drinking water, add a slice of lemon, lime, fresh mint leaves, or even pieces of ginger. Take a water bottle with you everywhere you go and refill it regularly. Sip on water throughout the day, even if you're not thirsty. Drinking carbonated water, in moderation, is also a way to meet your daily hydration goals. Soda, coffee, tea, and alcohol dehydrate the body. Even herbal teas act as mild diuretics. Limit your daily intake of these beverages.

Regular Movement – Move your body regularly. Chair yoga and low-impact exercises like swimming and biking can help you reach your weekly exercise quota, especially if walking isn't possible for you. Otherwise, brisk walking is an optimal way to stay healthy. A device that counts steps can motivate some folks to step up their walking game, especially in locations where walking isn't necessarily a part of daily life. When out shopping or on errands, park your car as far from the entrance as possible to log in extra steps. Walk around the block on your way to the mailbox. Whenever you get the chance, take the stairs.

Sleep Well – Try to get a good night's sleep. When possible, go to bed and wake up at a regular time. Reduce exposure to blue light rays, which negatively impact sleep hormone production, by purchasing blue light-blocking glasses and turning off your electronic devices at least an hour before bedtime. Avoid caffeine late in the day if you know you are sensitive to it, and limit your alcohol intake, which leads to poor quality sleep.

A Sharp Mind – Keep your brain active. Participate in engaging crossword puzzles or games that activate your mind. Study a new language, learn to play an instrument, or make some art. Creativity nourishes the mind. Some people find coloring in coloring books to be a very meditative activity. The brain is capable of creating new neural pathways throughout the lifespan, and you have the power to keep your mind agile through your daily activities and habits.

Take Care of Your Health – Schedule regular checkups at the doctor and dentist. You are the most familiar with your body's signals, so if you have an emergent health issue, don't wait to get it checked out. If you are experiencing a troubling sensation you've never had before, or you intuitively feel something is wrong with your body, listen to your gut and seek medical help. Don't hesitate to seek a second opinion, especially if you leave a doctor's appointment feeling your needs weren't heard or addressed.

Volunteer – Volunteering can be an incredible boost for your mental health and a way to combat solitude or feelings of disconnection. Though the objective is to help someone else, research reveals that the benefits of volunteering flow in both directions. It can be great to give back your time and energy to a cause that matters to you, connecting with the community and feeling like you're a part of something bigger than yourself. Doing so can reduce stress, fill you with intention, and increase your happiness and confidence. Studies have shown that rates of life satisfaction are higher among volunteers.

Exercise in a Group – There is something extraordinary about practicing yoga or movement with others. Research on synchronized group movement reveals that it promotes unity and cohesion among participants. If you have the resources to join a yoga, dance, tai chi, qigong, meditation, or any movement group class that piques your interest, try it! Check out discount rates at your local gym and apps such as MeetUp to see if there are local activities that you can join. Sometimes it's possible to do these activities at little or no cost.

Get Out into Nature – Time spent in nature boosts mental health. Whether in an accessible city park, a local forest, or a national park, breathing fresh air and focusing on the textures, sights, sounds, and ecosystems around you will calm your mind. Nature evokes innate observational skills that complement mindfulness practices. Even watching nature documentaries can alleviate the symptoms of depression and anxiety.

Overview

You can do all the yoga asanas you want; stretching, twisting, and pulling yourself into perplexing shapes on a beach at sunset, but if you're not breathing with intention, you're not doing yoga. Consciously connecting the breath and movement is the magic ingredient that transforms a stretching routine into a yoga practice. It links the mind and body, strengthens the balance system, profoundly relaxes the nervous system, and enhances the quality of presence as it prepares the body for meditation. Mastering your breath is just as important, if not more so, than learning yoga asanas.

The most common example of breathwork seen in Western culture is Lamaze breathing. TV shows and movies portray anecdotal and often humorous Lamaze breathing classes and births, with the mother coached through the technique before she screams bloody murder. Introduced to American obstetrics during the 1960s, breathwork and relaxation techniques marked a return to a more natural birthing approach. The science behind Lamaze is that it decreases pain perception and increases relaxation to reduce unnecessary medical interventions and promote safe and healthy births.

The ancient Indian yogis knew that breath was an indisputably powerful tool to influence, improve and maintain good health. They developed numerous breathing exercises known as pranayama (breath control). Pranayama consists of becoming conscious of the breath and moderating it through various cues and techniques. In this chapter, you'll learn the chair yoga go-to breathing pattern; in through the nose and out through the mouth, the diaphragmatic or belly, breath, and some easy pranayama for relaxation and nervous system regulation.

Anatomical Considerations

The diaphragmatic breath induces the parasympathetic nervous system, or the "rest and digest" function in the body, which decreases blood pressure, relaxes the heart and skeletal muscles, and increases nitric oxide, dilating blood vessels so oxygen-rich blood can circulate freely throughout the body. The increased amount of oxygen taken into the body during slow and steady diaphragmatic breathing counteracts stress hormones created during moments of anxiety, triggered so often in modern life. Diaphragmatic breathing also:

- ✿ Improves brain health
- ✿ Increases levels of focus and concentration
- ✿ Decreases emotional reactivity
- ✿ Improves emotional outlook

Until taught otherwise, most people breathe unconsciously. It isn't surprising, considering you don't need to think about your breath each time you take one; the autonomic nervous system manages that process. When people visualize taking a deep breath, the image that comes to mind might be an exaggerated breath through the mouth, hunched-up shoulders, and a puffed-out upper chest.

This quick and shallow breath triggers the sympathetic nervous system, or the "fight, flight, or freeze" response, which releases stress hormones. You automatically do it when frightened; your body floods with adrenaline to prepare you for a life-saving response. It may take time to unlearn what you define as a deep breath.

If you have ever observed a baby or young child about to sleep, you can see a clear example of the diaphragmatic, or belly, breath. They use their belly muscles to support diaphragmatic muscle function because their rib muscles have not yet fully developed. As we age, we often lose touch with our innate ability to breathe through the belly.

Nasal breathing optimizes the use of oxygen in the body. The nose is an intelligent filter that cleans, warms, and humidifies the air before it enters the lungs and makes possible our oldest sense, smell. Nasal breathing has a multitude of health benefits and is more beneficial for the body than mouth breathing. It increases oxygen levels in the blood compared to mouth breathing, strengthens the immune system, and improves lung volume.

If you have difficulty breathing through your nose, snore, or suffer from sleep apnea, take the time to investigate the underlying cause and seek treatment. Mouth breathing interrupts the body's ability to enter the deepest and most restorative sleep phases, leading to long-term fatigue and systemic dysregulation.

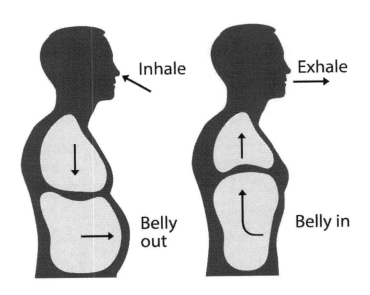

Inhale

Exhale

Belly out

Belly in

The respiratory system comprises the thoracic cavity or torso, the ribs, the thoracic muscles, the internal and external intercostal muscles, some neck, chest, and abdominal muscles, and the pelvic floor musculature. The diaphragm, a dome-shaped muscle located just below the lungs, at the bottom of the ribcage, is responsible for the ventilation of the body. It pumps air in and out of the lungs. When it pulls down, air enters the lungs as the belly, ribs, and lungs gently expand outwards. When the diaphragm pushes up, air exits the lungs as the belly, ribs, and lungs contract from the bottom up.

The parasympathetic nervous system activates during slowed respiration cycles and exhalation when the deepest lobes of the lungs contract and stimulate the vagus nerve, the largest cranial nerve that extends into the abdomen. Moderated by the breath, the vagus nerve controls heart rate, cardiovascular activity, breathing, digestion, and reflex actions like sneezing, coughing, and swallowing. It relays feedback about the body's level of relaxation to the brain for processing. Slow deep breaths are the anecdote to counteract the body's stress response.

Breathing exercises can help condition the pelvic floor muscles. Strong pelvic floor muscles aid in preventing pelvic organ prolapse. Pelvic organ prolapse is common among women, with nearly 50% experiencing some degree of prolapse in their lifetimes. More than 12% of women receive surgical treatment for this condition.

Symptoms of pelvic floor prolapse include:

- Incontinence
- Urinary leakage while coughing, laughing, or sneezing
- Feelings of heaviness or discomfort in the lower abdomen
- Feeling as though you're sitting on a ball
- Seeing or feeling a lump coming out of the vagina
- Pain or numbness during sex

There following factors can increase one's risk of prolapse:

- Menopause
- Having a hysterectomy
- Doing a job that requires heavy lifting
- Long-term strain to the bowels, including constipation or a chronic cough
- Pregnancy and childbirth, especially if you had an arduous birth, gave birth to multiple babies, or had a very large baby.

Prolapse is not dangerous; however, the frequency with which it occurs and the discomfort it can cause makes prevention and treatment a big priority. Symptoms can be relieved by a pessary, hormone replacement therapy, pelvic floor exercises, and in some cases, surgery.

Kegels

Kegels are the most well-known exercise for strengthening the pelvic floor muscles. You can identify these muscles by simply stopping the flow of urine mid-stream. However, don't habitually obstruct urination, as it can result in incomplete emptying of the bladder and lead to urinary tract infections. Also, avoid starting or stopping your urine stream by squeezing your pelvic floor muscles. Take care that you are not flexing surrounding muscles, including the abdomen, buttocks, or thighs.

Step 1: To begin, sit or lie down with an empty bladder.

Step 2: Take a gentle breath through your nose for a count of three.

Step 3: Visualize lifting and squeezing a marble with your pelvic floor muscles as you exhale through your mouth for a count of three.

Step 4: As you inhale, release your pelvic floor muscles for a count of three.

Step 5: As you exhale, squeeze your pelvic floor muscles for a count of three.

Step 6: Repeat 10 to 15 times.

Step 7: Work up to 3 reps a day.

You can safely integrate Kegels into the breathwork exercises described in this chapter and the exercises focusing on building abdominal strength in Chapter 9 during the exhalation phases. The important thing is to connect the exercise with your breath rhythm. When you inhale, relax your pelvic floor muscles. When you exhale, squeeze them.

The most common lung diseases are asthma, partial or complete lung collapse, bronchitis, lung infections, chronic obstructive pulmonary disease (COPD), lung cancer, fluid buildup, and a blocked lung artery. Studies indicate that breathing exercises can be an excellent complementary treatment for individuals with moderate to severe COPD and bronchial asthma.

Instructions

Contraindications – If you are pregnant or suffer from diabetes, high or low blood pressure, heart conditions, epilepsy, or vertigo, please consult your healthcare provider before performing these breathing exercises.

Stop if you feel discomfort or lightheadedness – Return to your normal breath and do not stand up. Dizziness can occur in beginners due to increased oxygen in the body, which causes blood vessels to dilate and lowers blood pressure, resulting in a temporary reduction of blood flow to the brain. It should subside with practice.

Never restrict or force your breath – The more you practice, the longer you can perform the exercises; eventually, your lung capacity will increase. Tune into your comfort level and move from one exercise to the next as you feel ready.

Keep count – If you have trouble monitoring your breath counts, don't hesitate to use your fingers to keep track.

Stay patient and focused on the journey – Over time, you'll notice the benefits of the practice.

What to Expect

These exercises provide a simple foundation to connect with the power of the breath. To prepare yourself for an enriching chair yoga practice, take your time learning these exercises. If you cannot breathe through your nose, in the meantime, focus on your breath awareness; pay attention to the rhythm of your breath as it enters and exits your mouth. In these directions, one breath comprises inhalation and exhalation.

Exercise 1 – Nasal Inhalation and Mouth Exhalation

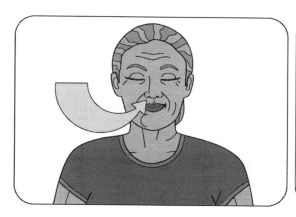 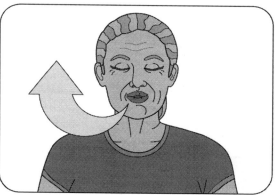

This exercise slows the breath rate. Practice inhaling slowly through the nose and elongating your exhalation as you seek to empty your lungs of air. It is physiologically impossible to do so; residual volume remains in the lungs even after a deep exhalation. Nevertheless, use this cue to get to the very bottom of your breath.

Step 1: Sit up tall on your chair in a stable position. Your legs should be hip-width apart, with your knees bent at a 90-degree angle stacked above your knees. Press your feet firmly against the floor and spread your toes as wide as possible.

Step 2: Squeeze your shoulder blades together to open the front of the chest. Lower your shoulders, and nod your chin slightly toward your chest to open the back of the neck. Relax your jaw.

Step 3: Place your left hand over your heart and your right hand above the belly button.

Step 4: Focus on the breath entering your nose and exiting through your mouth.

Step 5: Connect with your body's subtle movements, sensations, and sounds. You may feel your heart beating under your palm and your belly's gentle expansion and contraction as you breathe.

Step 6: When you're ready, take a slow and gentle inhalation through your nose, filling your lungs about three-quarters of the way.

    🌀   If you want to integrate Kegels, your pelvic floor muscles should relax as you inhale.

Step 7: As you exhale, purse your lips and breathe out very slowly until it feels like you have no more air left in your lungs. Keep going. You might be surprised by how long it takes!

        🌀 If you want to integrate Kegels, you can squeeze your pelvic floor muscles as you exhale.

Step 8: Repeat for 5 to 10 leisurely breaths, increasing the breath count with practice.

Step 9: Work up to 2 reps.

Once you feel comfortable with this exercise, you can experiment with pauses between the inhalation and the exhalation. Gently hold the air in your lungs for a few moments longer than usual before you begin your exhalation. After you exhale, do the same. Hold the void. Breath retention optimizes the benefits of this exercise.

Exercise 2 – The Diaphragmatic Breath

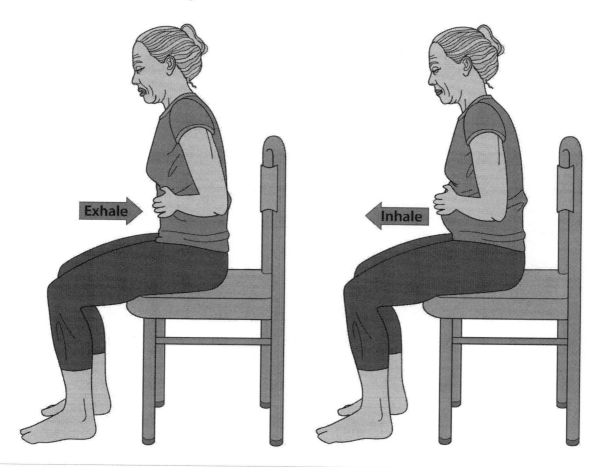

The diaphragm is like a bellows deep within your belly. Each inhalation and each exhalation is born from this muscle and then rises like a slow-motion wave to the top of the lungs. Your ribs will widen like an accordion. It's important to counteract teachings, especially for women, about "sucking it in" and constricting the abdominal muscles when breathing. Your connection to the diaphragmatic breath will strengthen each time you practice as you develop muscle memory.

Step 1: Sit up tall on your chair.

Step 2: Place your left hand over your heart and your right hand above the belly button.

Step 3: Take a normal breath through the nose.

Step 4: Purse your lips and exhale like you're blowing out a candle. You should feel the contraction of your diaphragm under your right hand. Visualize a balloon deflating. Keep exhaling until you have no breath left.

    🌀   If you want to integrate Kegels, you can squeeze your pelvic floor muscles as you exhale.

Step 5: Take a slow and deep breath through the nose. You should feel the expansion of your diaphragm under your right hand. Visualize a balloon inflating. Your belly and then your chest should rise as the breath moves upwards.

    🌀   If you want to integrate Kegels, your pelvic floor muscles should relax as you inhale.

Step 6: Repeat 2 more times.

Take your time playing with the number of breaths you take and the intensity of your exhalation to ensure your body gets accustomed to the amplified amount of oxygen in your blood. It can lead to lightheadedness initially as you work up to longer and deeper diaphragmatic breaths. As you gain confidence, slowly increase the number of deep and slow diaphragmatic breaths from 3 to 5 to 7 to 10, working up to 2 reps.

The directions indicate that you should feel your belly and chest expand as you inhale and contract as you exhale. Notice if this is true for you. It might not be! Becoming aware of this is the first step to rewiring your breath pattern. Some people have an intrinsic breathing pattern in which their belly and chest contract as they inhale and vice versa, and it can take working one-on-one with a breath coach in person or virtually to help you overcome it.

Exercise 3 – Breathing Aloud

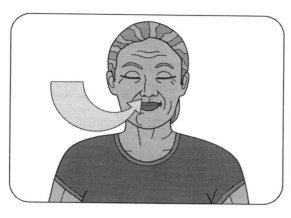 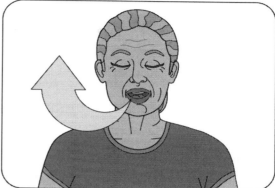

This straightforward exercise uses the power of sound to release bottled-up emotions, tension, and even pleasure. Incorporating sounds into your breath practice that reflect your emotional state can be liberating. If you're not practicing alone, give your family members or friends a heads-up that your yoga session will be vocal!

Step 1: Sit up tall on your chair.

Step 2: Place your left hand over your heart and your right hand above the belly button.

Step 3: Connect with the movement under your palms. You may feel your heart beating or your belly rumbling. Stay present with this.

Step 4: Begin with three slow and steady diaphragmatic breaths.

Step 5: Then, consciously inhale through the nose. When you exhale through the mouth, add an audible sigh, "ah," or "vroo" sound. It can be a quiet, loud, happy, or frustrated sound – whatever feels suitable for you now. Feel free to let out a howl if you're feeling frisky or if it's the full moon!

Step 6: Repeat 5 to 7 times.

Do this breath when you feel like you've been holding something in. Sometimes, emotions get stuck when we're not able to vocalize them. It can be refreshing to free your voice and invite its unhindered expression.

Exercise 4 – The Box Breath

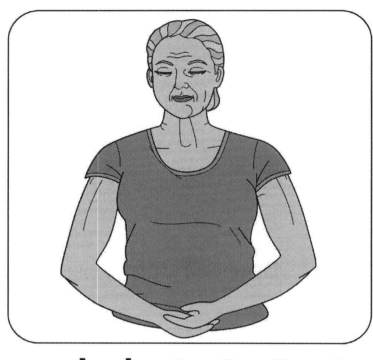

inhale 1...2...3...4

hold 1...2...3...4

exhale 1...2...3...4

rest 1..2..3...4

Once you've mastered the diaphragmatic breath, combine it with this box breath technique. Box breath is a powerful tool that you can use to combat stress and anxiety. It's straightforward and incredibly effective.

Do this exercise in 4 counts, or modify that number according to your breathing rhythm. For example, some might find a count of 3 or 7 more comfortable. The important thing is keeping it equal.

Step 1: Sit up tall on your chair.

Step 2: Inhale through the nose for four counts.

Step 3: Hold your breath for four counts.

Step 4: Exhale through the mouth for four counts.

Step 5: Hold the exhale (don't breathe in) for four counts.

Step 6: Repeat 5 to 10 times.

Exercise 5 – The 4-8-7 Technique

Another powerful relaxation method is the 4-8-7 technique. It will naturally calm your mind and body. You can do it whenever you feel anxious or before bed to help you fall asleep.

Step 1: Sit up tall on your chair.

Step 2: Inhale through your nose for 4 seconds.

Step 3: Hold your breath for 7 seconds.

Step 4: Purse your lips and exhale gently through your mouth for 8 seconds

Step 5: Repeat this breathing cycle up to 4 times.

Exercise 6 – Alternate Nostril Breathing

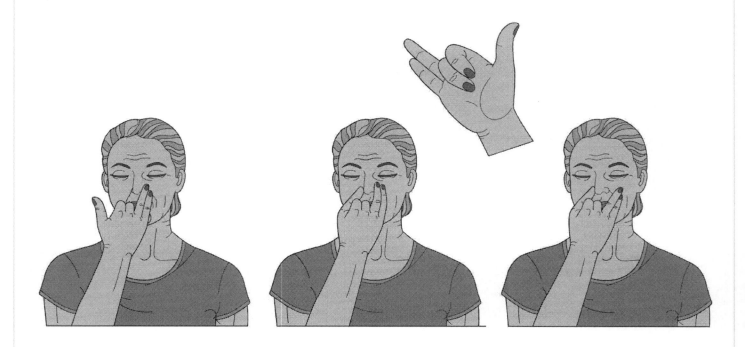

Alternate nostril breathing slows the breath rate considerably. You're filling both lungs with air drawn from just one nostril and releasing it slowly through the opposite nostril. If you have a deviated septum or a clogged nostril, you can practice this hands-free and visualize the breath moving through the blocked side. This pranayama always begins and ends on the left side.

Step 1: Sit up tall on your chair.

Step 2: Gently close the right nostril with the right thumb.

Step 3: Inhale slowly through the left nostril.

Step 4: Close the left nostril with your ring or pinky finger.

Step 5: Lift your thumb and exhale through the right nostril.

Step 6: Inhale through the same side, the right nostril.

Step 7: Close the right nostril with your thumb.

Step 8: Exhale through your left nostril.

Step 9: Inhale through the same side, the left nostril.

Step 10: Close the left nostril with your ring or pinky finger.

Step 11: Lift your thumb and exhale through the right nostril.

Step 12: Inhale through the same side, the right nostril.

Step 13: Close the right nostril with your thumb.

Step 14: Exhale through your left nostril.

Start with 5 to 10 breaths and slowly increase the number as you master the technique. Keep your breath soft and gentle.

Overview

This gentle and comprehensive warmup series invites you to reconnect with your body from head to toe. It's good to begin any workout with a warmup, and chair yoga is no different. Warming up prepares the muscles for action, increases heart rate, and stimulates blood flow, allowing more oxygen to reach your muscles, thus reducing your risk of injury.

Instructions

Now is the perfect time to start cultivating good vibes! It's possible to reorient the patterns of the mind with thoughtfulness and attention. Positive affirmations can help you improve your mood and boost your self-esteem.

Before you start your chair yoga routine, experiment with setting a positive intention. It can be as effortless as a one-word or one-sentence affirmation you say to yourself, representing the quality of energy you wish to amplify and invite into this time you've carved out for yourself.

For example, if you've had a stressful day, this is your opportunity to say that you wish to relax. You might choose the word "relaxation." If you are an incessant self-critic, or maybe something is going on in your life that you're having difficulty coming to terms with, you might select "acceptance" as your word. Sometimes acceptance isn't even possible, in which case you can give yourself permission not to accept what's happening and have compassion for that. You can also work with mantras from the Hindu tradition or prayers from your spiritual or religious background.

Here are some more examples:

- Trust
- Peace
- Kindness
- I love myself
- I am healing
- I am grateful for my body
- I meet myself where I am
- I honor and care for myself

These exercises are easy to remember, and you can do them before starting any chair yoga workout. Reconnect with your body and give them a go!

Exercise 1 – Grounding

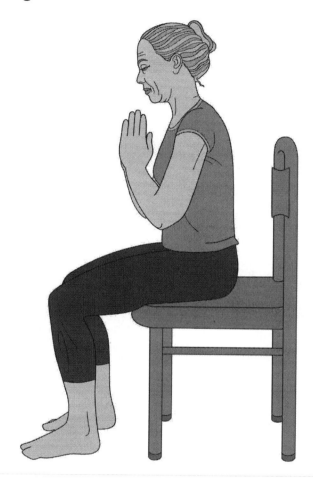

This grounding warmup invites you to connect with your body and breath to bring focus and intentionality to your practice. It is your go-to position to start any seated chair yoga exercise unless otherwise specified.

Step 1: Sit up tall on your chair in a stable position. Your legs should be hip-width apart, with your knees bent at a 90-degree angle stacked above your knees. Press your feet firmly against the floor and spread your toes as wide as possible.

Step 2: Squeeze your shoulder blades together to open the front of the chest. Lower your shoulders, and nod your chin slightly toward your chest to open the back of the neck. Relax your jaw.

Step 3: Bring your hands together in a prayer position before your heart and smile.

Step 4: Close your eyes, and scan your body and mind for any tension you might be carrying.

Step 5: Take a few moments to reconnect with your breath. Consciously begin to release any tension as you exhale.

Step 6: Once you feel grounded and calm, set a simple positive intention or affirmation for your workout.

Exercise 2 – Neck "U" Rotation

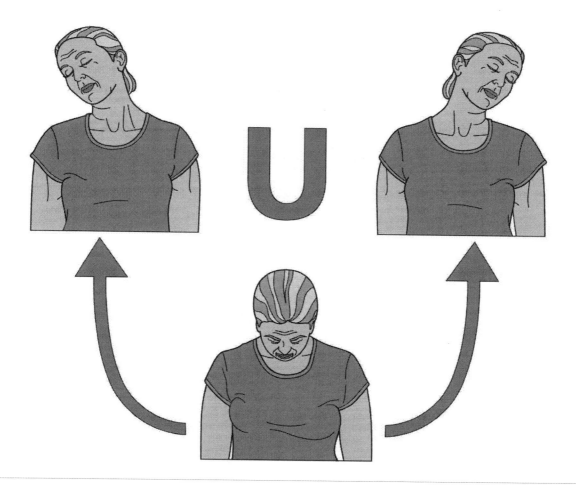

This exercise warms up the muscles at the back of the neck.

Step 1: Sit up tall on your chair.

Step 2: Inhale through the nose as you roll your chin in a gentle arc from your chest to a point above the left shoulder. Exhale through the mouth as you roll your chin to the center.

Step 3: Inhale as you roll your chin gently in an arc, a "U" shape, from the center of your chest to a point above the right shoulder. Only go as far as is comfortable. Exhale through the mouth as you drop your chin to your chest.

Step 4: Repeat 5 to 10 times on each side.

Exercise 3 – Arm Rotations

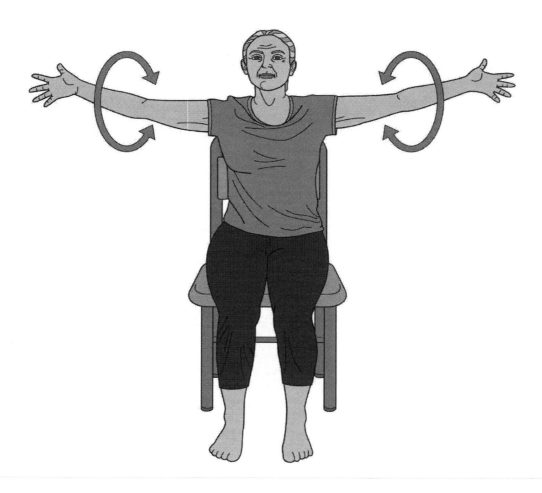

Arm rotations are great for warming up the shoulder joints.

Step 1: Sit up tall on your chair.

Step 2: Inhale through the nose and extend your arms to either side. Exhale through the mouth as you rotate your arms in tight circles 10 to 20 times.

Step 3: You can gradually widen the arc of your circles and then tighten them as you come to stillness.

Step 4: Repeat circles going in the opposite direction.

Exercise 4 – Hand Clenches

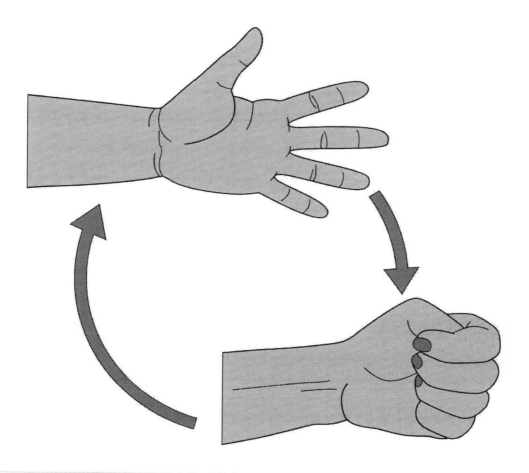

Hand clenches encourage blood flow to the hands and the wrists and help release tension, which can be especially beneficial after a long day at work.

Step 1: Sit up tall on your chair.

Step 2: Extend your arms in front of you.

Step 3: Spread your fingers wide, then squeeze them toward your palms.

Step 4: Repeat 10 to 15 times, working up to 2 reps.

Exercise 5 – Sweeping Arms Flow

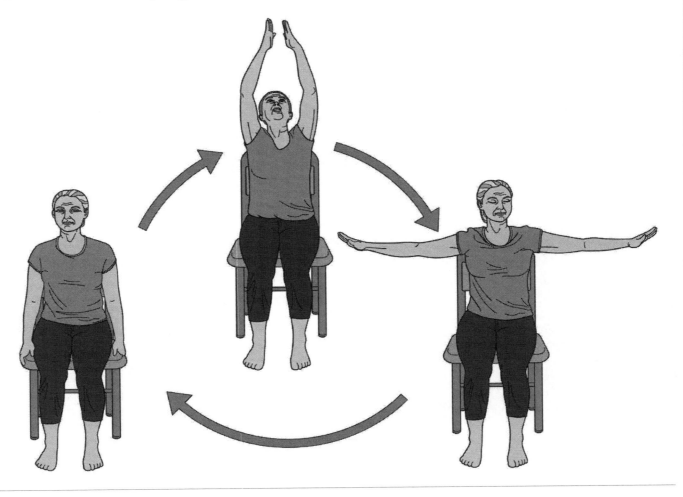

This exercise energizes the arms, shoulders, and upper back.

Step 1: Sit up tall on your chair.

Step 2: Inhale through the nose as you sweep your arms out and then up to the sky.

Step 4: Exhale through the mouth as you lower your arms.

Step 5: Repeat this flow for at least 5 to 7 slow breaths, working up to 2 reps.

Exercise 6 – Seated March

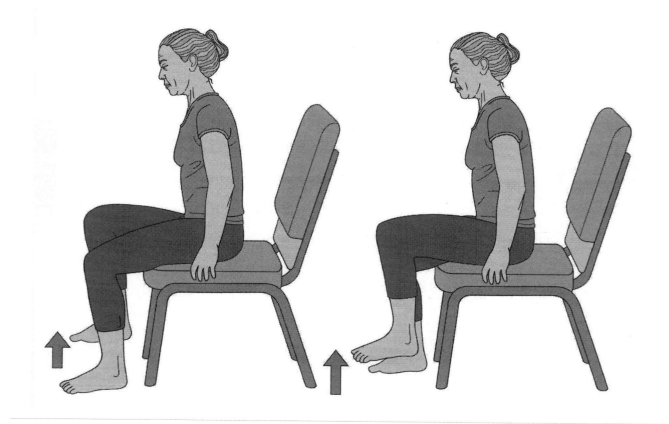

Seated march targets and strengthens the hip flexors and legs. It's a great, low-impact exercise for those with knee replacements.

Step 1: Sit up tall on your chair.

Step 2: Alternate lifting one knee at a time. You can also bend your elbows at a 90-degree angle and add energetic arm swings to accompany your march.

Step 3: Lift your knees 15 to 20 times, working up to 2 reps.

Exercise 7 – Ankle Rotations

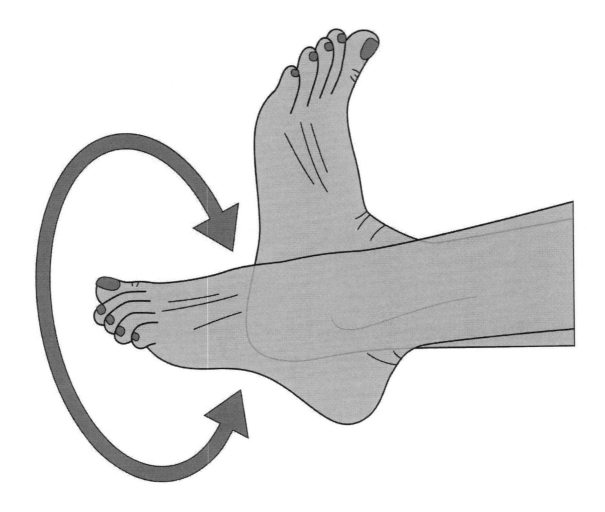

Ankle rotations are excellent to make sure your ankles stay flexible and supple.

Step 1: Sit up tall on your chair.

Step 2: Lift one foot at a time and circle 10 to 15 times in one direction.

Step 3: Switch directions.

Step 4: After you finish, shake, shake, shake your feet!

Exercise 8 – Integrate

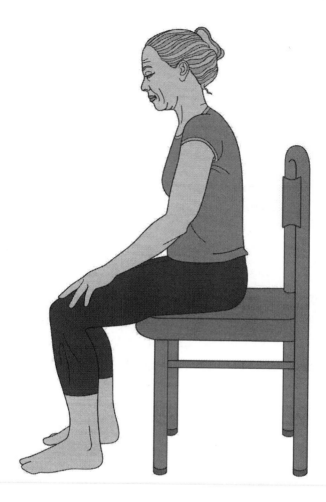

This closing exercise is an opportunity to integrate the benefits of the practice.

Step 1: Sit up tall on your chair.

Step 2: Bring your hands to rest on your thighs.

Step 3: Close your eyes, and reconnect with your breath.

Step 4: Smile gently, take a few moments to observe your feelings after the practice, and thank yourself for caring for your body and mind.

CHAPTER 5 | BALANCE

Overview

Unless you've experienced dizziness or vertigo, you may have yet to spend much time thinking about the body's spatial awareness operating system, the balance system. Yet an estimated 35% of individuals aged 40 and above in the United States have vestibular (inner ear) dysfunction that can cause symptoms of dizziness. Women are up to three times more likely than men to be affected by it. In addition to heightened anxiety and depression, the significant consequence of balance issues is an increased fall risk. Falls can result in fractures, broken bones, and long-term recovery and rehabilitation, impacting an individual's ability to lead a mobile and independent life.

Anatomical Considerations

The balance system consists of the eyes, the inner ear (a mysterious structure resembling a seashell nestled close to the brainstem), and the joints and muscles of the body, which send real-time signals about your body's location in space and time to various parts of the brain. Once synthesized, this information relays back as motor output to the skeletal muscles and eyes, which makes it possible to move without anticipating your next step.

Proper balance depends on the brain coordinating and harmonizing these signals with the least interference possible. When any of the components of the balance system are compromised, the ability to process spatial information can suffer. Loss of hearing, vision, or sensation in the legs are common conditions that can negatively impact a person's balance.

What is the Difference Between Dizziness and Vertigo?

Dizziness is commonly described as follows:

- ෧ feeling off balance or unsteady, faint or lightheaded, woozy or giddy
- ෧ feeling like you're walking on a soft surface or mattress
- ෧ feeling drunk without imbibing alcohol or standing in a boat in choppy water

Vertigo is characterized by a spinning sensation even when still. Vertigo is referred to as a fear of heights in popular culture, but the fear of heights is called acrophobia. Of course, vertigo could result as a side effect of acrophobia, but they are not the same.

Vertigo can be described in the following ways:

- ⟳ Feeling as though you're spinning, or your surroundings are spinning around you
- ⟳ Feeling like you're falling or pushed from behind
- ⟳ Feeling a revolving sensation or that you're swaying
- ⟳ Feeling like you're on a merry-go-round

Essential questions to ask yourself:

- ⟳ Does my vision become blurred?
- ⟳ Do I lose my balance and fall?
- ⟳ Do I feel as though I'm falling?
- ⟳ Do I feel like I'm moving, even when standing still?
- ⟳ Do I feel as though the room is spinning around me?
- ⟳ Do I feel unsteady?
- ⟳ Do I feel lightheaded or like I might faint?

If you answered yes to any of the questions above, do not hesitate to investigate what is causing it. Take your concerns to a medical professional. Dizziness is a symptom that has numerous underlying causes, so it may take some in-depth investigation to determine the root of your symptoms.

Some common underlying causes of dizziness and vertigo include certain medications, migraine headaches, alcohol, benign positional vertigo (BPV), Meniere's Disease, anxiety disorders, stress, heat stroke, excessive exercise, anemia, motion sickness, a sudden drop in blood pressure, loss of blood volume, dehydration, heart disease, and ear infection.

When to seek emergency medical attention? Get help if you experience dizziness or vertigo accompanied by chest pain, nausea, vomiting for extended periods, headache, neckache, blurred vision, high fever, hearing loss, difficulty speaking, droopiness of the eye or mouth, loss of consciousness, or a head injury. Although rare, dizziness or vertigo can also be caused by stroke, multiple sclerosis, brain tumors, or other brain disorders.

Feeling dizzy and having difficulty with your balance can be scary. You may notice certain things trigger your dizziness. Keep a journal of what you eat and drink and what activities precede these experiences. The following tips can help reduce dizziness.

Hydrate – Drink 8 to 10 glasses of water every day. Drink a glass first thing in the morning. Coffee and black tea have high caffeine levels, activating the sympathetic nervous system and the body's stress response. Try switching to green tea, which has less caffeine and contains antioxidants that benefit your body's cells. Consider cutting back or quitting alcohol and smoking completely.

Eat well – Take measures to reduce your daily salt intake. You might be surprised by how much salt your favorite foods contain. For dizziness relief, the ancient wisdom of Indian Ayurveda prescribes a light, bland, simple diet with no spices. Eat fresh citrus fruits, poppy seeds, dates and raisins, and green vegetables such as kale or broccoli.

Bodywork – A certified upper cervical spine chiropractor can work wonders for those with dizziness. The vestibular system is located in the upper cervical vertebrae region, so adjusting this area can create more space for the inner ear fluid to drain. Acupuncture can be beneficial by stimulating blocked energy points in the body to regulate and calm the nervous system. Regular massages and even self-massage can help release stress.

Supplements – Some supplements can improve symptoms of dizziness and vertigo. They include vitamin D, calcium, ginger, ginkgo biloba, L-lysine, and lemon bioflavonoids.

Instructions

Your balance system will benefit from these exercises. They focus on strengthening the visual and vestibular systems. They fortify the muscles around the eyes, engage the inner ear, and improve hand-eye coordination. Slowly, you will train your balance system to create new neural connections to improve sensory processing.

Practice chair yoga barefoot and walk without shoes or slippers as often as possible. When you walk barefoot, more surface area on the bottom of your feet touches the ground, sending valuable data about your spatial position back to the brain. This information is also known as proprioception or kinesthesia.

Always listen intently to your body. Ease yourself into practice. If any exercise causes dizziness, stop immediately. Take a break until you feel normal, and either try again or move to the next exercise. Take extra precautions if you have an elevated fall risk. You'll need a ball for exercise 8. If you don't have a yoga ball, don't worry, a tennis ball or even a rolled-up sock can work.

Exercise 1 – Grounding

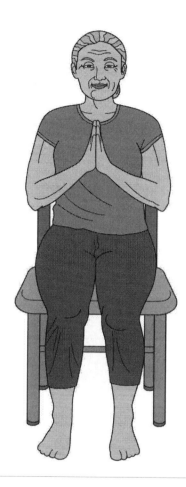

This grounding warmup invites you to connect with your body and breath to bring focus and intentionality to your practice.

Step 1: Sit up tall on your chair in a stable position. Your legs should be hip-width apart, with your knees bent at a 90-degree angle stacked above your knees. Press your feet firmly against the floor and spread your toes as wide as possible.

Step 2: Squeeze your shoulder blades together to open the front of the chest. Lower your shoulders, and nod your chin slightly toward your chest to open the back of the neck. Relax your jaw.

Step 3: Bring your hands together in a prayer position before your heart and smile.

Step 4: Close your eyes if it doesn't cause dizziness, and scan your body and mind for any tension you might be carrying.

Step 5: Take a few moments to reconnect with your breath. Consciously begin to release any tension as you exhale.

Step 6: Once you feel grounded and calm, set a simple positive intention or affirmation for your workout.

Exercise 2 – Head and Eyes Same Direction

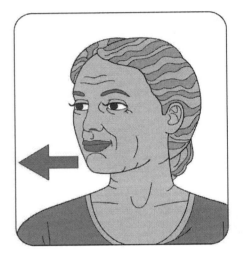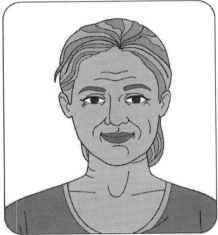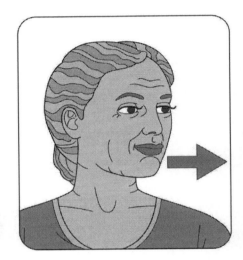

Step 1: Sit up tall on your chair.

Step 2: Find a point in the mid-distance and focus your gaze there.

Step 3: Slowly turn your head and eyes in tandem to the right.

Step 4: Return to the center, and repeat on the left side.

Step 5: Repeat 5 to 10 times, working up to 2 reps.

Exercise 3 – Eyes Side to Side

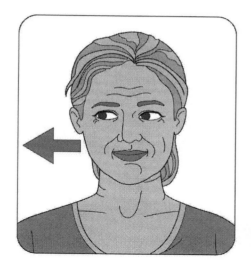 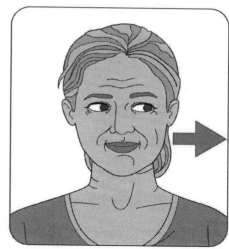

Step 1: Sit up tall on your chair.

Step 2: Find a point in the mid-distance and focus your gaze there.

Step 3: Without moving your head, slowly look to the right, as far as is comfortable. Bring your gaze back to the center. Repeat on the left side.

Step 4: Repeat 5 to 10 times, working up to 2 reps.

Exercise 4 – Eyes Up and Down

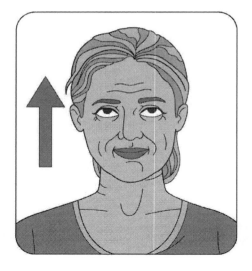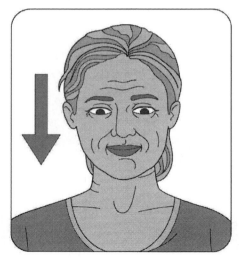

Step 1: Sit up tall on your chair.

Step 2: Find a point in the mid-distance and focus your gaze there.

Step 3: Without moving your head, slowly look upwards as far as is comfortable. Bring your gaze back to the center. Slowly look down as far as is comfortable, again, without moving your head. Bring your gaze back to the center.

Step 4: Repeat 5 to 10 times, working up to 2 reps.

Exercise 5 – Finger Focus

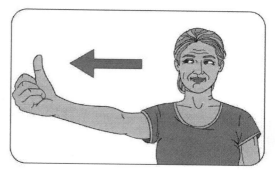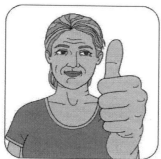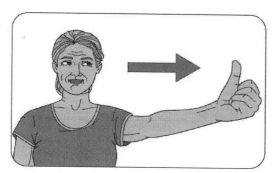

Step 1: Sit up tall on your chair.

Step 2: Extend your right thumb about 1 foot before you.

Step 3: Focus your gaze on your thumb.

Step 4: Without moving your head, follow your thumb with your eyes as you slowly move the thumb to the right of your field of vision and then back to the center.

Step 5: Extend your left thumb about 1 foot before you.

Step 6: Without moving your head, follow your thumb with your eyes as you slowly move the thumb to the left of your field of vision and then back to the center.

Step 7: You can practice this with your thumb held out at various distances.

Step 8: Repeat 5 to 10 times, working up to 2 reps.

Exercise 6 – Alternate Eye Covers

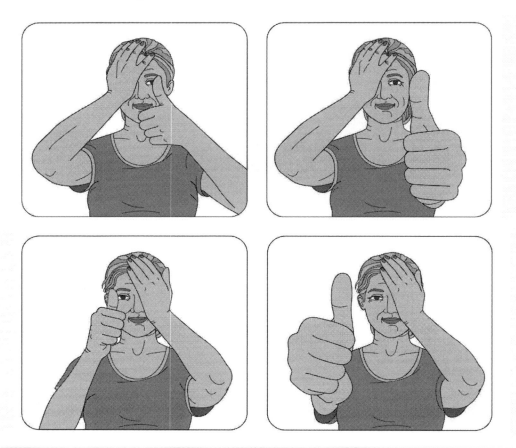

Step 1: Sit up tall on your chair.

Step 2: Cover your right eye with your right hand.

Step 3: Extend your left arm in front of you and stick your thumb out.

Step 4: Focus your gaze on your thumb.

Step 5: Stay focused on your thumb as you slowly bring your thumb close to your eye and back it away again, repeating 5 to 10 times.

Step 6: Cover the left eye and repeat the exercise on the opposite side.

Step 7: Work up to 2 reps

Exercise 7 – Figure 8 Circles

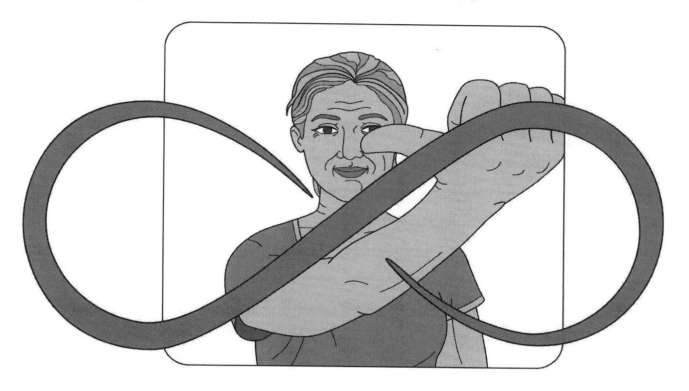

Step 1: Sit up tall on your chair.

Step 2: Find a point in the mid-distance and focus your gaze there.

Step 3: Hold your right arm straight ahead.

Step 4: Stick out your thumb as though you are hitchhiking.

Step 5: Make a figure 8 gesture with your hand as you focus on your thumb.

Step 6: Repeat this exercise 5 to 10 times in one direction.

Step 7: Repeat on the opposite side.

Step 8: Work up to 2 reps.

Exercise 8 – Ball Toss Above Head

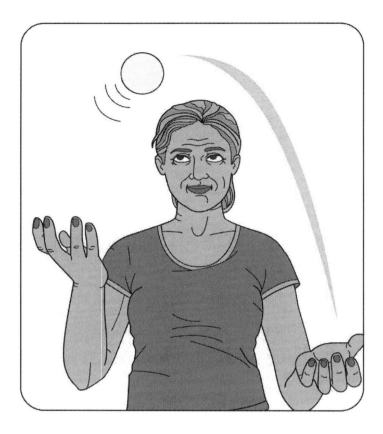

This exercise will help you to improve your hand/eye coordination.

Step 1: Sit up tall on your chair.

Step 2: Toss the ball from one hand to another while watching it.

Step 3: As you gain confidence, toss the ball above eye level to increase hand-eye coordination.

Step 4: Continue this for several minutes, building up to more extended periods as your coordination improves.

Exercise 9 – Integrate

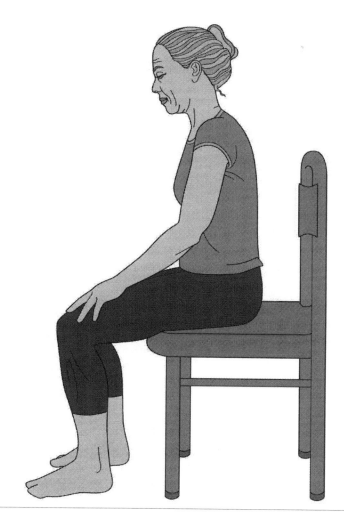

This closing exercise is an opportunity to integrate the benefits of the practice.

Step 1: Sit up tall on your chair

Step 2: Bring your hands to rest on your thighs.

Step 3: Close your eyes, and reconnect with your breath.

Step 4: Smile gently, take a few moments to observe your feelings after the practice, and thank yourself for caring for your body and mind.

Overview

Technology use negatively influences posture. Just observe anyone hunched over their smartphone. Jobs that require sitting for long periods working on a computer are also culprits of poor posture. The neck and shoulders bear much of the brunt of the modern slouch. Chests are concave; shoulders are hunched; necks jut forward, carrying the heavy load of the brain. Consequently, the back, neck, and shoulder muscles get overstretched and fatigued, while the chest muscles become underused and foreshortened. You might feel an accumulation of tension between the neck and shoulders, resulting in diminished shoulder mobility, tender points, and knots.

Anatomical Considerations

The cervical spine is the uppermost region of the spine located in the neck. It protects the spinal cord, provides blood flow to the brain, and supports the head's weight. It is a complex structure composed of vertebrae, bones, discs, muscles, tendons, ligaments, and nerves. It makes a wide range of motion possible.

The most common injuries to the cervical spine in older adults are fractures resulting from falls. If you experience tingling, numbness, weakness, or an inability to move your head due to a fall, seek medical attention immediately. Other common injuries include sprains, pinched nerves, arthritis, spondylosis (wear and tear of the cervical vertebrae and cartilage), and whiplash. Symptoms of injury or damage to this region include pain, swelling, and reduced range of motion.

Do you feel a dull ache at the outside edge of your shoulder that has grown progressively more painful over time? Are daily activities a struggle: putting on a shirt, retrieving objects from a high shelf, pulling weeds, or throwing a ball around with your grandkids? These could be symptoms of rotator cuff tendonitis.

The shoulder joint has the most mobility and the least structural stability of all the joints. The rotator cuff comprises a group of four muscles and tendons that keep the ball joint in place. They begin at the inner edge of the shoulder blade, cross the shoulder joint, and attach at the upper arm bone, making arm movement possible. There is an elevated risk for rotator cuff tears among people who participate in repetitive sports, such as basketball, golf, tennis, baseball, and yoga. Tears from trauma can happen in any contact sport, like ice hockey, lacrosse, and football.

If you have chronic or acute pain in your shoulder joint/s, please consult a medical professional to diagnose and identify the source of this pain, as injuries to the various muscles of the rotator cuff may require different treatments.

Good workstation ergonomics can help you prevent shoulder and neck pain. Position your computer screen directly in your line of sight, reduce blue light emissions from your screen, and use blue light-blocking glasses. Adjust your chair height so that your knees fold at a 90-degree angle, adjust the height of your desk so your elbows rest at 90 degrees, and use a wrist pad. Sit tall at the edge of your chair with both feet on the ground.

Chair yoga can be a life-changing practice for those with sedentary desk jobs. Start doing these simple stretches from this chapter throughout your workday. Take the stairs at every opportunity and go for a walk on your break. Advocate for an office culture that actively supports wellness activities and movement.

Other sore shoulder and neck pain remedies include:
- Acupuncture
- Regular massages
- Experiment with different pillows
- Learn self-massage techniques and apply sore muscle balm
- Apply warm compresses to sore muscles

Instructions

Your neck and shoulders will benefit from these stress and tension relief exercises. They'll help you open the shoulder girdle (the connective tissue around the shoulder) and strengthen the muscles for a more stable shoulder joint. You will need a yoga strap or alternative to complete the eighth exercise.

Exercise 1 – Grounding

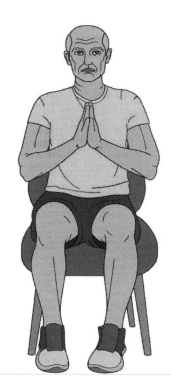

This grounding warmup invites you to connect with your body and breath to bring focus and intentionality to your practice.

Step 1: Sit up tall on your chair in a stable position. Your legs should be hip-width apart, with your knees bent at a 90-degree angle stacked above your knees. Press your feet firmly against the floor and spread your toes as wide as possible.

Step 2: Squeeze your shoulder blades together to open the front of the chest. Lower your shoulders, and nod your chin slightly toward your chest to open the back of the neck. Relax your jaw.

Step 3: Bring your hands together in a prayer position before your heart and smile.

Step 4: Close your eyes, and scan your body and mind for any tension you might be carrying.

Step 5: Take a few moments to reconnect with your breath. Consciously begin to release any tension as you exhale.

Step 6: Once you feel grounded and calm, set a simple positive intention or affirmation for your workout.

Exercise 2 – Up and Down Neck Rolls

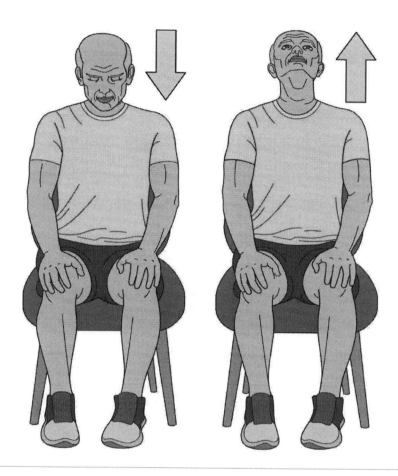

This exercise gently stretches the muscles at the front and back of the neck.

Step 1: Sit tall on your chair.

Step 2: Inhale and lift your chin to the sky.

Step 3: Exhale your chin back down to the chest.

Step 4: Repeat 5 to 10 times, working up to 2 reps.

Exercise 3 – Center to Side Neck Rotation

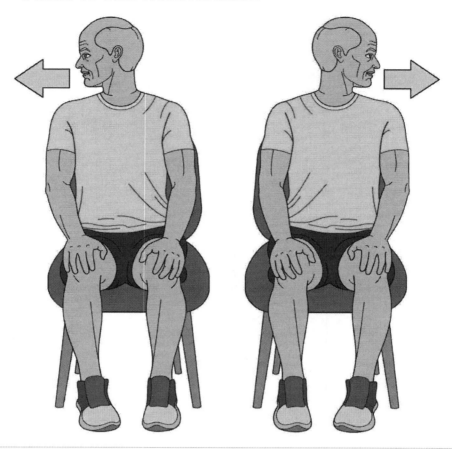

This stretch tones the muscles on the sides of the neck and gives the cervical spine a gentle twist.

Step 1: Sit tall on your chair.

Step 2: Inhale gently through the nose.

Step 3: Exhale through your mouth as you turn your head smoothly to the right.

Step 4: Inhale back to the center.

Step 5: Exhale through your mouth as you turn your head smoothly to the left.

Step 6: Inhale back to the center.

Step 7: Repeat 5 to 10 times, working up to 2 reps.

Exercise 4 – Side Neck Stretch

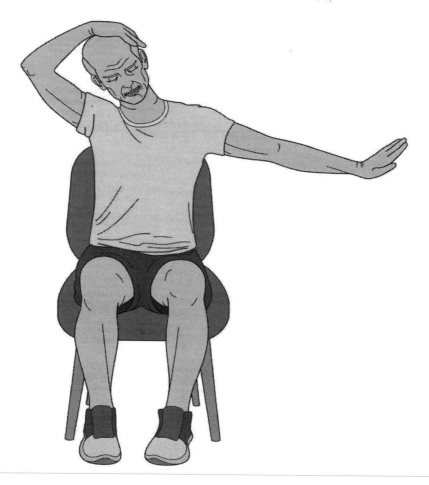

This simple seated neck stretch helps release tightness in the shoulders, neck, and upper back.

Step 1: Sit tall on your chair.

Step 2: Tilt your head toward your left shoulder, placing your left hand above your right ear and pressing down as you gently stretch the right side of your neck.

Step 3: Return your head to the center and take three slow breaths before continuing.

Step 4: Tilt your head toward your right shoulder, placing your right hand above your left ear, pressing down gently as you stretch the left side of your neck.

Step 5: Hold each side for 5 to 7 gentle inhalations through the nose and out through the mouth, working up to 2 repetitions.

Exercise 5 – Alternate Shoulder Shrugs

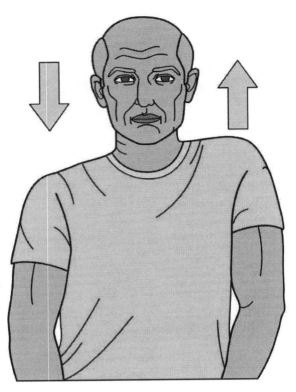

Alternate shoulder shrugs help boost energy in the body and work the areas where we store a lot of tension.

Step 1: Sit tall on your chair.

Step 2: Inhale as you slowly shrug your right shoulder up.

Step 3: Exhale as you drop it back down.

Step 4: Inhale as you slowly shrug your left shoulder up.

Step 5: Exhale as you drop it back down.

Step 6: Repeat 10 to 15 times on each side

Exercise 6 – Hands-On Shoulder Rolls

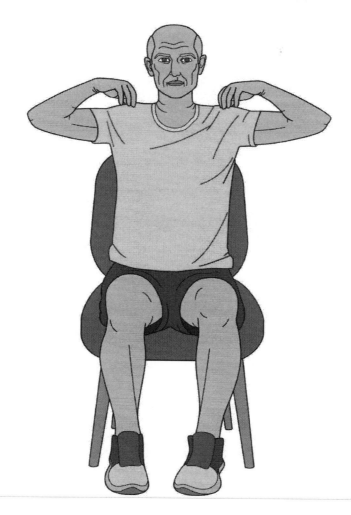

You can do this exercise to warm up the shoulders and upper back.

Step 1: Sit tall on your chair.

Step 2: Inhale as you lift your arms out to the sides. As you exhale, bring your fingertips to your shoulders.

Step 3: Begin to circle in one direction. Circles can be large or small.

Step 4: Pause and reverse.

Step 5: Circle 10 to 15 times in each direction, working up to 2 repetitions.

Exercise 7 – Overhead Shoulder Stretch

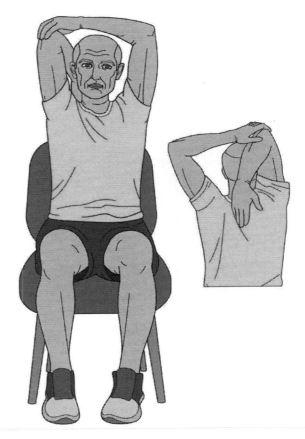

This beginner-level stretch pose brings mobility and flexibility to the shoulders.

Step 1: Sit tall on your chair.

Step 2: Inhale and raise your right arm.

Step 3: Exhale, bend your right arm at your elbow and position your right hand on the center of your upper back.

Step 4: Inhale and grasp your right elbow with the left hand.

Step 5: Gently pull your elbow towards your head to deepen the stretch.

Step 6: Stay here for 5 to 7 slow breaths.

Step 7: Repeat on the opposite side.

Exercise 8 – Rotator Cuff Stretch

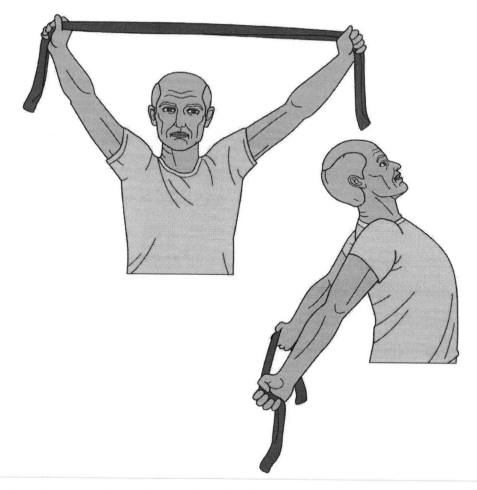

You'll need a strap or strap alternative for this stretch. This incredible shoulder stretch opens up the chest for better posture.

Step 1: Sit tall on your chair.

Step 2: Grasp a strap before you, holding it more than shoulder-width apart.

Step 3: Lift the strap above your head and guide it up and over your head, then behind your back. Extend your hands as wide as necessary so that this movement is pain-free and doesn't force your range of motion. Go only as far as comfortable.

Step 4: Repeat 5 to 10 times, working up to 2 repetitions.

Exercise 9 – Integrate

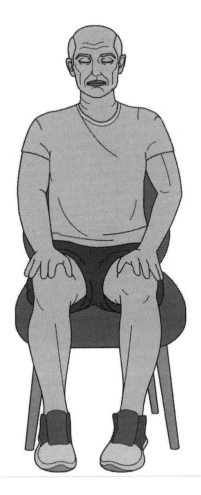

This closing exercise is an opportunity to integrate the benefits of the practice.

Step 1: Sit up tall on your chair.

Step 2: Bring your hands to rest on your thighs.

Step 3: Close your eyes, and reconnect with your breath.

Step 4: Smile gently, take a few moments to observe your feelings after the practice, and thank yourself for caring for your body and mind.

C H A P T E R 7 | HANDS & ARMS

Overview

Yoga is excellent for stretching and toning the hands and arms. Fine motor coordination of the fingers and hands makes it easy to do precise movements such as holding a pen or a spoon, buttoning a button, or typing on the computer. If you are a writer, a musician, an artist, or anyone whose profession or hobby relies on deft hand movements, you know that aches and pains in this region of the body can quickly derail your job and passions. Strengthening your arm muscles makes everyday activities like lifting and reaching for objects easier. You have the option to incorporate weights into this chair yoga routine. Strength training improves heart health and increases bone density and muscle tone.

Anatomical Considerations

The brain region dedicated to controlling the hands is vast, which hints at the importance of their function in our species. The hands are an intricate structure that consists of 27 bones with the ability to articulate their 27 joints in highly nuanced ways. The hand has 34 muscles and more than 100 tendons and ligaments.

The most common hand injuries include tendonitis, repetitive strain injury, carpal tunnel syndrome, fractures, muscle strains, sprains, dislocation, and osteoarthritis. Chronic aches and pains can indicate an overuse injury.

The arms have 24 muscles which make it possible to complete seven different actions: flexion, extension, internal and external rotation, abduction (lifting the arm away from the body), adduction (drawing the arm back to the body), and circumduction (arm circles). The upper arm only has five muscles, while the lower arm has 19. The forearm muscles are highly specialized to control the function of the wrist and hands.

Common arm injuries include bursitis, tendonitis, sprains, dislocations, nerve problems, fractures, and osteoarthritis.

Tweak your home and office ergonomics to avoid common hand and wrist injuries when using a computer or tablet. Ensure that your wrists are level when you work, that they aren't angled upwards as you type, and that they're not resting against a hard, compressive surface all day. It can lead to muscle strain, decreased blood flow to the hands, and nerve compression. When using a mouse, ensure your wrist isn't bent away from the thumb, which puts undue stress on the wrist joint.

In addition, make sure that your elbows are at a 90-degree angle as you work. Arms flexed more than this put pressure on blood vessels and nerves. Please seek a diagnosis from a medical professional for any unusual or unexplained pain in your arms, wrists, hands, or fingers.

Instructions

There are many benefits to doing exercises for your hands and arms. For starters, it can help improve your grip strength, which can be handy for everyday activities like opening jars or carrying groceries. Additionally, strengthening your hands and arms can help prevent injuries, alleviate pain in these areas and improve your overall upper body strength. Don't neglect them! You will need a yoga ball or alternative for the fourth exercise. You can add light hand weights to exercises 5, 6, and 7.

Exercise 1 – Grounding

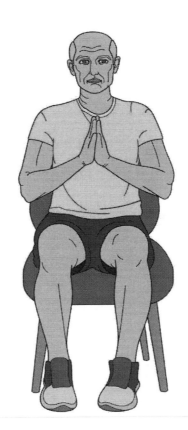

This grounding warmup invites you to connect with your body and breath to bring focus and intentionality to your practice.

Step 1: Sit up tall on your chair in a stable position. Your legs should be hip-width apart, with your knees bent at a 90-degree angle stacked above your knees. Press your feet firmly against the floor and spread your toes as wide as possible.

Step 2: Squeeze your shoulder blades together to open the front of the chest. Lower your shoulders, and nod your chin slightly toward your chest to open the back of the neck. Relax your jaw.

Step 3: Bring your hands together in a prayer position before your heart and smile.

Step 4: Close your eyes, and scan your body and mind for any tension you might be carrying.

Step 5: Take a few moments to reconnect with your breath. Consciously begin to release any tension as you exhale.

Step 6: Once you feel grounded and calm, set a simple positive intention or affirmation for your workout.

Exercise 2 – Wrist Joint Rotation

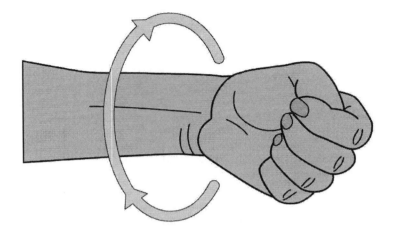

This exercise helps warm up the wrist joints.

Step 1: Sit tall on your chair.

Step 2: Extend your arms in front of you, shoulder-width apart.

Step 3: Create a fist with your hand.

Step 4: Rotate your wrists clockwise 10 - 15 times

Step 5: Repeat, circling your wrists counterclockwise 10 - 15 times.

Exercise 3 – Wrist Extension

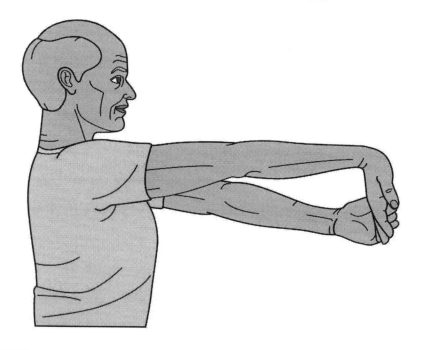

Wrist extensions stretch out the forearm extensors, the muscles which make gripping possible.

Step 1: Sit tall on your chair.

Step 2: Extend your left hand in front of you, with your palm facing the sky.

Step 3: With your right hand, gently press the fingers of the left hand toward your body. You should feel this stretch from the underside of your wrist to the elbow.

Step 4: Hold here for 5 to 7 deep inhalations through the nose and exhalations through the mouth.

Step 5: Repeat on the opposite side.

Step 6: Work up to 2 reps.

Exercise 4 – Ball Squeeze

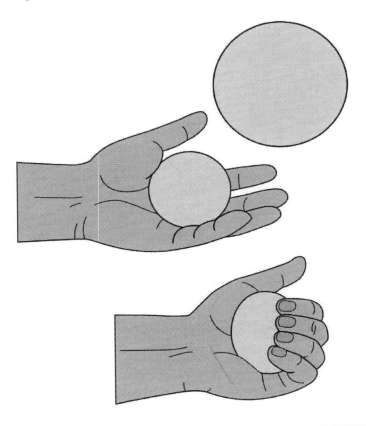

This exercise increases grip strength by conditioning the wrist, fingers, and thumb flexors. The repetitive motion also improves fine motor skills.

Step 1: Sit tall on your chair.

Step 2: Take your yoga ball in your hand. If you have two, put one in each hand; otherwise, just alternate.

Step 3: Squeeze your ball tight for 5 to 10 seconds.

Step 4: Work up to 5 reps.

Exercise 5 – Seated Fist Punches

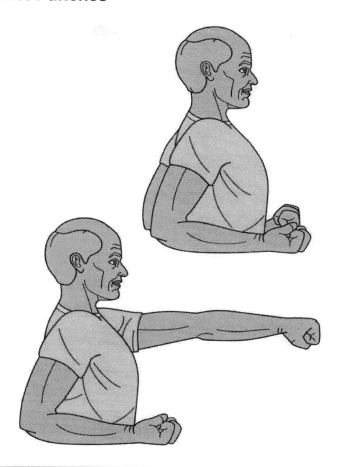

Seated fist punches condition the entire upper body, especially the biceps and triceps in the arms. Add light weights if it feels comfortable for you.

Step 1: Sit tall on your chair.

Step 2: In a comfortable seated position, bring your arms to your sides, your elbows bent at a 90-degree angle, and your hands in a fist.

Step 3: Start throwing some slow punches one arm at a time. Rotate your fist to the center as you extend your arm so that the top of your fist faces the sky. As you retract your arm, rotate it so your knuckles face the sky.

Step 4: Start with one round of 10 to 15 punches, and slowly work up to 2 or 3 reps.

Exercise 6 – Seated Cactus Arms Flow

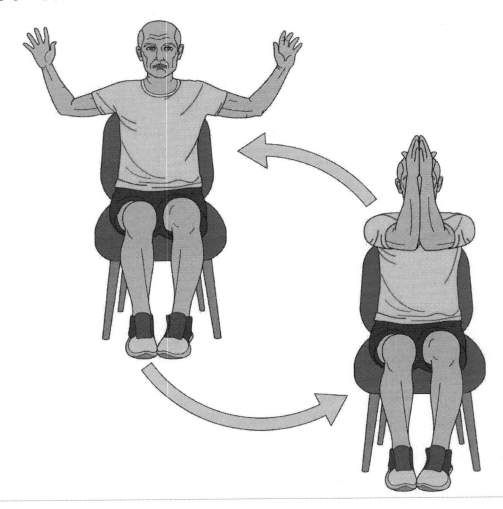

This exercise will increase strength and flexibility in the upper back, chest, neck, arms, and shoulders. Add light weights if it feels comfortable for you.

Step 1: Sit tall on your chair.

Step 2: Extend your arms to either side with your elbows bent at a 90-degree angle, fingers pointed to the sky.

Step 3: Draw your forearms together in front of you.

Step 4: Inhale as you open your arms, and exhale as you bring your arms together again.

Step 5: Repeat 10 to 15 times, and slowly work up to 2 reps.

Exercise 7 – Goddess Pose with Cactus Arms

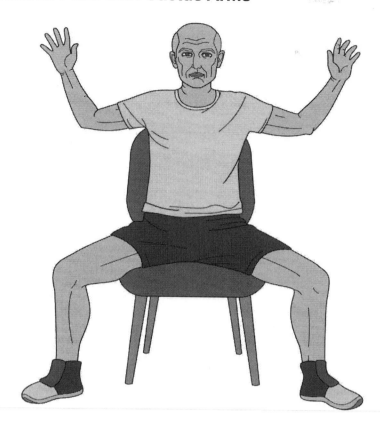

This isometric pose activates the shoulders, arms, biceps, and triceps. Add light weights if it feels comfortable for you.

Step 1: Sit tall on your chair.

Step 2: Position your legs wider than hip-width apart, with your toes angled slightly outward.

Step 3: Lift your arms to either side, bend your elbows at a 90-degree angle, and point your fingers to the sky.

Step 4: Squeeze your shoulder blades together and lift through your chest.

Step 5: Press your feet into the floor, elongate your spine, and tuck your chin gently toward your chest.

Step 6: Hold here for 5 to 7 slow breaths in through the nose and out through the mouth, working up to 2 reps.

Exercise 8 – Seated Eagle Arms

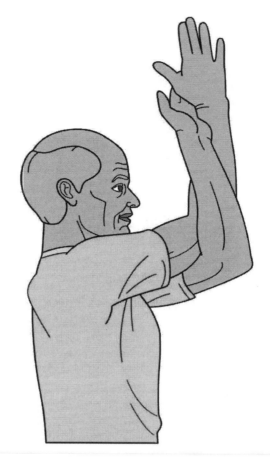

Seated Eagle arms targets the shoulders, back, and neck and helps stretch arthritic elbows, wrists, and fingers.

Step 1: Sit tall on your chair.

Step 2: Extend both arms in front of you.

Step 3: Place your left elbow over your right elbow.

Step 4: Bend both arms at the elbows at a 90-degree angle.

Step 5: Press the backs of your hands together.

Step 6: Hold here for 5 to 7 slow breaths through the nose and out through the mouth.

Step 7: Release and repeat on the opposite side.

Exercise 9 – Integrate

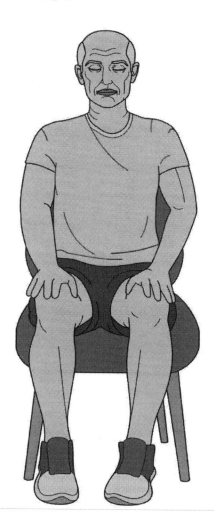

This closing exercise is an opportunity to integrate the benefits of the practice.

Step 1: Sit up tall on your chair.

Step 2: Bring your hands to rest on your thighs.

Step 3: Close your eyes, and reconnect with your breath.

Step 4: Smile gently, take a few moments to observe your feelings after the practice, and thank yourself for caring for your body and mind.

Overview

Who has not felt a twinge in the back after digging in the garden all afternoon, shoveling snow, or lifting a heavy box? Muscle strains and ligament sprains are the most common types of back injury. Poor posture, falls, and sports injuries can contribute to back injuries. They can occur suddenly or over time. If you suffer from back pain, chair yoga has a variety of exercises that will be helpful for you to get back on track and find relief.

Anatomical Considerations

The mid-back is called the thoracic spine. It comprises twelve thoracic vertebrae that begin at the base of the neck and end roughly near the bottom of the ribcage. It makes a slight "C" shape. The rhomboid muscles connect the mid-back to the inside edge of the shoulder blades, making it possible to rotate the torso, draw the shoulder blades together, pull, throw, and raise our arms.

Discomfort in this area can be caused by bad posture, sitting for too long, and injuries, overstretching, or torn muscles.

Additional causes of middle back pain include:

- ⑤ Spinal stenosis (spinal canal narrowing)
- ⑤ Arthritis of the spine
- ⑤ Herniated, ruptured, or degenerated discs

Osteoporosis can also cause middle back pain. Women over the age of 50 are especially prone to osteoporosis, so scheduling regular bone density scans is essential.

The lower back is called the lumbar region of the spine and comprises five sturdy vertebrae. It curves to make a slight backward "C" shape. The latissimus dorsi, the "lats," is the broadest and most powerful muscle in the back. It originates at the lower back and sweeps upwards in a wide "V" shape. It crosses the shoulder joints and attaches to the upper arm bones. The lats stabilize the back and make it possible to raise your arms above your head, do pull-ups, row, swim, and breathe. Strong lats facilitate good posture.

Chronic lower back pain lasts more than three months. It can be attributed to lumbar herniated disks, degenerative disk disease, facet joint dysfunction, sacroiliac joint dysfunction, spinal stenosis, spondylolisthesis (a slipped vertebrae), osteoarthritis, spinal curvature, acute fractures, compression fractures or vertebral dislocations. Don't hesitate to get to the root cause of your back pain if it is a chronic issue. Many underlying causes can be effectively treated and healed.

Chair yoga can help you release tightness in the lower back and strengthen your back muscles to enhance stamina and posture. Yoga is an excellent antidote for back pain. Learn about the ergonomics of lifting with good posture. Exercise regularly, build strength and flexibility, keep a healthy weight, and quit smoking and drinking to decrease your likelihood of back injuries.

Instructions

This mid- and upper-back chair yoga routine targets the back muscles and spine to increase flexibility and mobility. Some exercises focus on opening up the front of the chest to counteract poor posture. Spinal twists promote flexibility and range of motion in the spine. Individuals with osteopenia or osteoporosis of the spine should avoid spinal twists. Avoid forward bends and lowering your head below your heart if you have unmanaged high blood pressure. Forward bends can be modified by placing your forearms on your thighs and staying upright or by placing blocks below your hands and keeping your head level.

Exercise 1 – Grounding

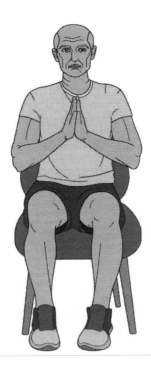

This grounding warmup invites you to connect with your body and breath to bring focus and intentionality to your practice.

Step 1: Sit up tall on your chair in a stable position. Your legs should be hip-width apart, with your knees bent at a 90-degree angle stacked above your knees. Press your feet firmly against the floor and spread your toes as wide as possible.

Step 2: Squeeze your shoulder blades together to open the front of the chest. Lower your shoulders, and nod your chin slightly toward your chest to open the back of the neck. Relax your jaw.

Step 3: Bring your hands together in a prayer position before your heart and smile.

Step 4: Close your eyes, and scan your body and mind for any tension you might be carrying.

Step 5: Take a few moments to reconnect with your breath. Consciously begin to release any tension as you exhale.

Step 6: Once you feel grounded and calm, set a simple positive intention or affirmation for your workout.

Exercise 2 – Overhead Arm Stretch

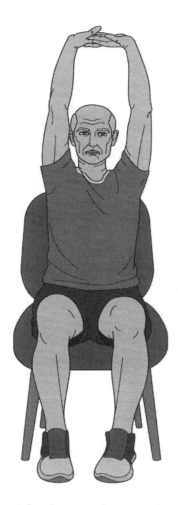

The overhead arm stretch is great for improving posture by lengthening the spine and strengthening the torso muscles.

Step 1: Sit tall on your chair.

Step 2: Inhale as you raise your arms above your head until your palms touch.

Step 3: Interlace your fingers, and rotate your palms to the sky.

Step 4: Stay here for 5 to 7 deep breaths through the nose and out through the mouth, working up to 2 reps.

Exercise 3 – Cat-Cow

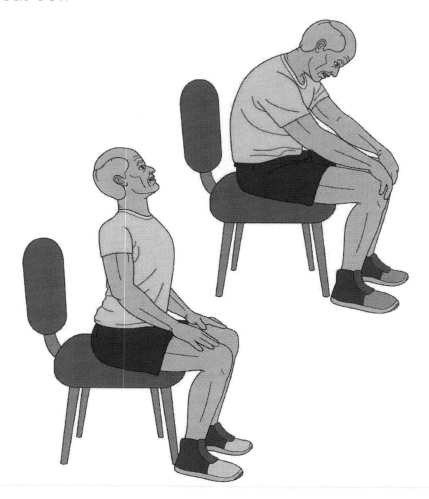

Cat-cow mobilizes and rejuvenates the spine.

Step 1: Sit tall on your chair.

Step 2: Place your hands on your thighs.

Step 3: Inhale through the nose as you arch your back by squeezing your shoulder blades together, opening your chest, and gently lifting your chin to the sky.

Step 4: Exhale through the mouth as you round your mid and upper back and lower your chin to your chest.

Step 5: Repeat 5 to 10 times, working up to 2 reps, following the rhythm of your breath.

Exercise 4 – Cobra

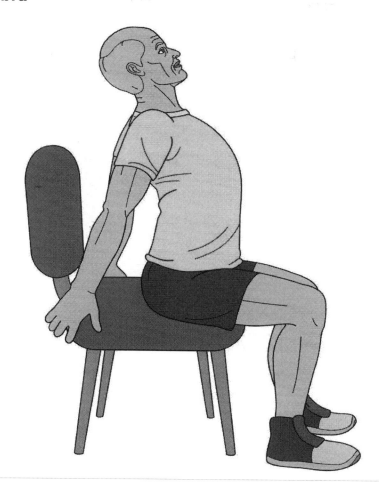

This pose targets the mid-back, the upper back, and the chest.

Step 1: Sit tall on your chair.

Step 2: Gently reach behind you to grasp the back of the chair.

Step 3: Squeeze your shoulder blades together, and open the front of your chest. Gently lift your chin to the sky.

Step 4: Stay here for 5 to 7 deep breaths through the nose and out through the mouth, working up to 2 reps.

Exercise 5 – Seated Twist

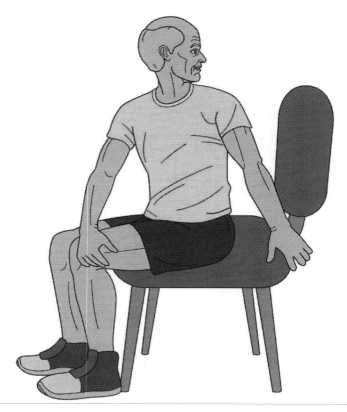

Seated twist targets the neck, hips, shoulders, and back muscles. Twists are basic movements that, if practiced regularly, preserve the normal range of motion of the spine. Those with osteopenia or osteoporosis of the spine should avoid it.

Step 1: Sit tall on your chair.

Step 2: Grasp the back of the chair behind you with your right hand.

Step 3: Place your left hand on your right knee.

Step 4: Begin the twist by turning your head to gaze over your right shoulder. Your torso will follow. You can deepen the twist by pressing your left hand against your right knee.

Step 5: Stay here for 5 to 7 gentle breaths through the nose and out through the mouth.

Step 6: Reverse sides and repeat, working up to 2 reps.

Exercise 6 – Sage Marichi

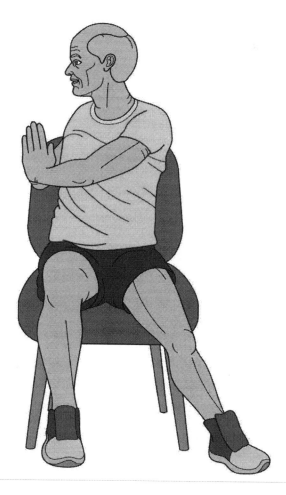

Your lower back and hamstring muscles will benefit from this gentle pose. Those with osteopenia or osteoporosis of the spine can modify it by avoiding step 4.

Step 1: Sit tall on your chair.

Step 2: Extend your left leg so your heel touches the ground.

Step 3: Bring your hands to the prayer position before your heart.

Step 4: Slowly twist your torso to the right and hold.

Step 5: Take 5 to 7 slow breaths through the nose and out through the mouth.

Step 6: Reverse sides and repeat, working up to 2 reps.

Exercise 7 – Goddess Side Stretch

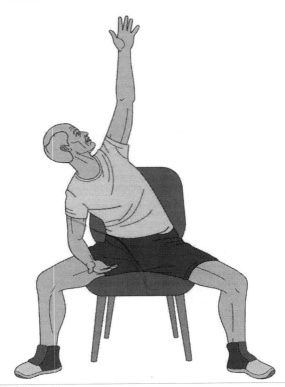

This pose releases tightness and stiffness in the shoulders and back.

Step 1: At the edge of the chair, open your legs wide and point your feet out to either side at a 45-degree angle.

Step 2: Bend slightly to the right and rest your right forearm on your right thigh.

Step 3: Lift your left arm to the ceiling.

    🌀   To adjust this pose, place your left hand on your hip, or lift it as comfortably as possible. Focus on keeping your chest and left shoulder open.

Step 4: You can gaze up to the sky, straight ahead, or at the floor, depending on how your neck feels.

Step 5: Stay here for 5 to 7 slow inhalations through the nose and exhalations through the mouth.

Step 6: Reverse sides and repeat, working up to 2 repetitions.

Exercise 8 – Wide Legged Forward Bend

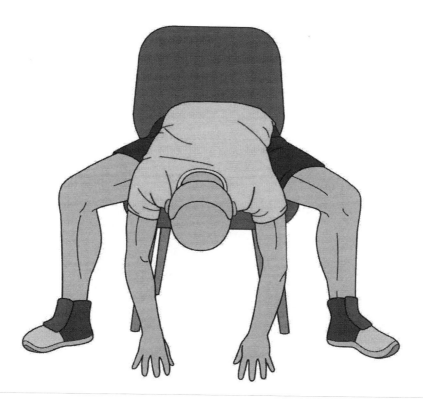

This pose is a good stretch for the inner thighs, the joints of the hips, knees, spine, neck, shoulders, and body parts that can collect stress and tension. Don't lower your head below your heart if you have uncontrolled high blood pressure.

Step 1: At the edge of the chair, open your legs wide and point your feet out to either side at a 45-degree angle.

Step 2: Inhale through your nose as you lift your arms above your head.

Step 3: Exhale through your mouth as you hinge forward at the hips, keeping a flat back as you gently lower your torso to a horizontal position as your place your hands on the ground.

   ✿   To adjust this pose, place blocks below your hands or lower your torso slightly and support yourself with your hands on your thighs.

Step 4: Stay here for 5 to 7 deep breaths in through the nose and out through the mouth, working up to 2 repetitions

Exercise 9 – Integrate

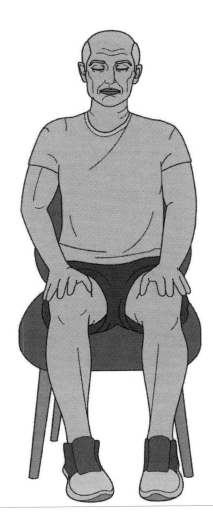

This closing exercise is an opportunity to integrate the benefits of the practice.

Step 1: Sit up tall on your chair.

Step 2: Bring your hands to rest on your thighs.

Step 3: Close your eyes, and reconnect with your breath.

Step 4: Smile gently, take a few moments to observe your feelings after the practice, and thank yourself for caring for your body and mind.

CHAPTER 9 | ABDOMINALS

Overview

The abdominals make it possible to laugh, sneeze, cough, and complete essential bodily functions. They unite the upper and lower parts of the body, and many of our everyday activities require abdominal activation, including standing, sitting, bending, lifting, reaching, turning, and singing, to name a few.

Abdominal muscle exercises improve pelvic, lower back, and hip function by creating more stability in the body's center. Better posture and balance prevent falls and injuries. Four out of five adults will experience lower back pain, and practicing chair yoga is a fantastic way to strengthen the abdominal muscles, reducing the likelihood of injury.

Anatomical Considerations

The abdominal muscles consist of five different muscles which perform various functions. The two vertical muscles keep internal pressure in the abdomen and help hold the organs in place. Three flat muscles in the stomach stabilize the trunk and assist with maintaining abdominal pressure.

Common abdominal injuries include muscle strains. Commonly called a muscle "pull," a muscle strain is when the muscle or tendon gets stretched too far. Severe strains feature partial or even complete tears of the tissue. They can result from overuse injuries (a repetitive action that results in gradual pain), a traumatic injury during sports, or even an activity such as lifting something heavy with poor body mechanics. Symptoms include tenderness, localized soreness, swelling, and even difficulty breathing.

A hernia is a common abdominal injury in which an internal organ pushes through a weak spot in the muscle. It can sometimes present as a bulge or bump, aches, heaviness, or pain at the injury site. If you have trouble moving, breathing, sleeping, sitting, or walking due to pain in your abdominals, or if you see a bulge or bump in your abdomen or groin, seek medical assistance to investigate the underlying cause.

Chapter 3 investigates pelvic organ prolapse, risk factors, and treatments. Please refer to the Kegels exercise, which you can integrate into the abdominal exercises in this chapter. To help prevent undue stress on the pelvic floor muscles, especially if you are at risk for or have experienced pelvic organ prolapse in the past, you can engage your pelvic floor muscles using Kegels during the exhalation phase of these exercises.

Instructions

Chair yoga abdominal exercises are a great way to improve your overall health and fitness by strengthening your core muscles and improving your posture, balance, and stability. Additionally, abdominal workouts can help reduce your risk of back pain and injury and improve your athletic performance. You can enjoy these benefits and more by incorporating these abdominal exercises into your routine.

Exercise 1 – Grounding

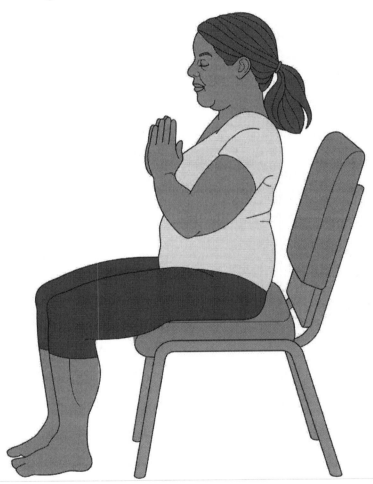

This grounding warmup invites you to connect with your body and breath to bring focus and intentionality to your practice.

Step 1: Sit up tall on your chair in a stable position. Your legs should be hip-width apart, with your knees bent at a 90-degree angle stacked above your knees. Press your feet firmly against the floor and spread your toes as wide as possible.

Step 2: Squeeze your shoulder blades together to open the front of the chest. Lower your shoulders, and nod your chin slightly toward your chest to open the back of the neck. Relax your jaw.

Step 3: Bring your hands together in a prayer position before your heart and smile.

Step 4: Close your eyes, and scan your body and mind for any tension you might be carrying.

Step 5: Take a few moments to reconnect with your breath. Consciously begin to release any tension as you exhale.

Step 6: Once you feel grounded and calm, set a simple positive intention or affirmation for your workout.

Exercise 2 – Seated Torso Circles

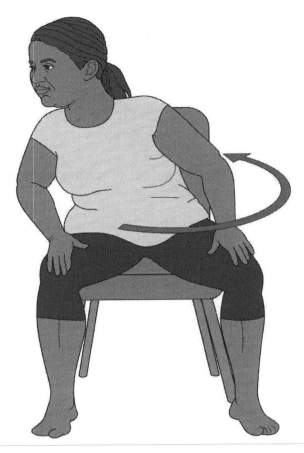

Seated torso circles benefit the psoas (the deepest core muscle), the lower back, and the pelvis.

Step 1: Sit tall on your chair.

Step 2: Place your hands on your thighs.

Step 3: Inhale gently through the nose and out through the mouth.

Step 4: Slowly rotate your torso clockwise 10 to 15 times. Start with small circles and gradually widen them. You can lift your arms to either side if this feels good to you.

Step 5: Slowly come back to the center.

Step 6: Repeat with counterclockwise rotations.

Exercise 3 – Alternate Arm and Leg Extensions

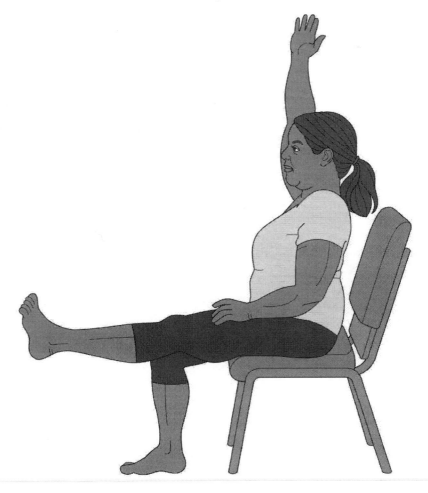

This pose builds strength and increases stability in the abdominal region.

Step 1: Sit tall on your chair.

Step 2: Take a gentle inhalation through your nose as you raise your right arm overhead and extend your left leg straight before you.

Step 3: Exhale through the mouth as you lower your arm and leg at the same time.

Step 4: Repeat with the opposite arm and leg until you've completed 5 to 10 sets on both sides.

Step 5: Work up to 2 reps.

Exercise 4 – Staff Pose

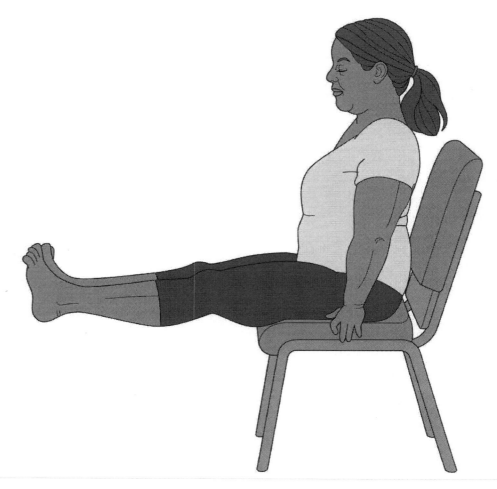

This exercise engages the abdominals and promotes good posture.

Step 1: Find a comfortable seat in the center of the chair. With an elongated spine and open heart, grasp the seat on either side of you with your hands.

Step 2: Engage your belly and as you inhale through the nose, lift your legs at the same time.

Step 3: Keep your legs straight and parallel to the ground. Engage your quadriceps and flex your toes towards your torso. Exhale through your mouth.

Step 4: Take 5 to 7 slow breaths in through the nose and exhale through the mouth.

Step 5: Work up to 2 reps.

Exercise 5 – Boat Pose

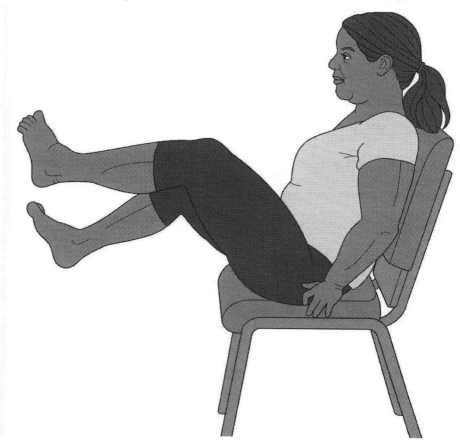

You are guaranteed to feel the burn with this pose! It strengthens the abs, energizes the body, aids digestion, reduces back pain, and encourages restful sleep.

Step 1: Find a stable seat in the center of the chair.

Step 2: Grasp the sides of the chair for stability.

Step 3: Lean back slightly.

Step 4: Keep your abdominal muscles tight as you lift your knees towards your chest. Ensure that you feel balanced here.

Step 5: Slowly lift your ankles and extend your legs.

Step 6: Stay here for 5 to 7 gentle breaths through the nose and out through the mouth.

Step 7: Slowly work up to 2 to 3 reps.

Exercise 6 – Chair Pose

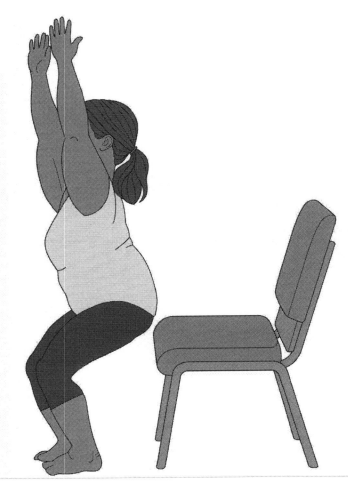

You'll strengthen the lower back, abdominal muscles, glutes, and knees in this pose.

Step 1: Sit tall on your chair.

Step 2: With a straight back, hinge forward slightly from the hips.

Step 3: Take a deep inhalation through the nose as you squeeze your belly muscles and lift from your hips to a standing position.

Step 4: Exhale through your mouth and bend your knees like you will sit down but hover above the chair seat instead.

Step 5: Inhale as you raise your arms above your head and shoulders.

Step 6: Exhale through the mouth.

Step 7: Stay here for 5 to 7 gentle breaths, working up to 2 reps.

Step 8: Return to a seated position.

Exercise 7 – Goddess Side Stretch

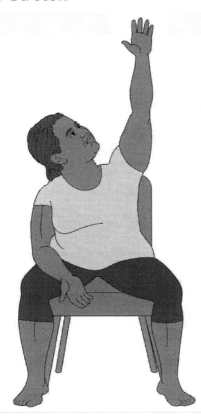

This exercise builds lower body strength as it improves overall stability in the body. It releases tightness and stiffness of the shoulders and back.

Step 1: Sit tall, open your legs wide, and point your toes out at a 45-degree angle.

Step 2: Place your right forearm on the top of your right thigh.

Step 3: Lift your left arm toward the ceiling and raise your gaze to your left palm.

   ✺   You can also look straight forward or at the ground to adjust this pose.

Step 4: Hold this pose for 5 to 7 gentle breaths through the nose and out through the mouth.

Step 5: Come back to the center. Repeat on the other side, working up to 2 reps.

Exercise 8 – Seated Downward Facing Dog

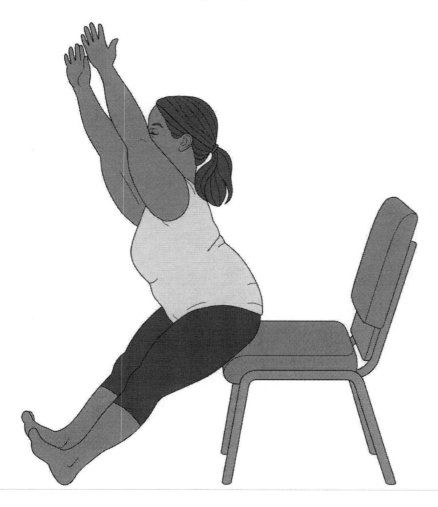

This exercise engages the abdominal muscles and lengthens the spine and hamstrings.

Step 1: Sit tall on your chair.

Step 2: With your legs hip-width apart, straighten your legs with your heels touching the ground. You should feel a slight stretch at the back of your knees.

Step 3: Inhale gently through the nose as you lift your arms shoulder-width apart above your head with your palms facing each other.

Step 4: Exhale through the mouth and slowly hinge forward from your hips into a balanced posture.

Step 5: Stay here for 5 to 7 slow inhalations through the nose and out through the mouth.

Exercise 9 – Integrate

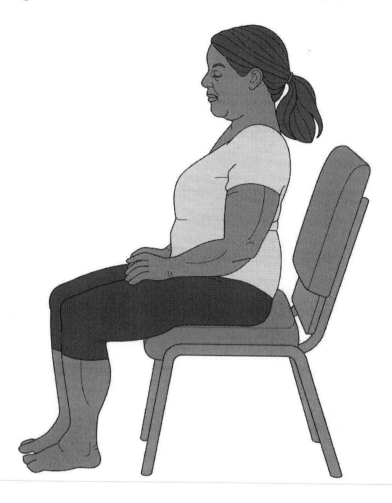

This closing exercise is an opportunity to integrate the benefits of the practice.

Step 1: Sit up tall on your chair.

Step 2: Bring your hands to rest on your thighs.

Step 3: Close your eyes, and reconnect with your breath.

Step 4: Smile gently, take a few moments to observe your feelings after the practice, and thank yourself for caring for your body and mind.

CHAPTER 10 | HIPS

Overview

The hip joints are stable and weight-bearing, making the movement of the lower extremities possible. A sedentary lifestyle can lead to tight hip muscles, causing sciatica and pain in the lower back and gluteal region. Chair yoga for the hips will help you release tension in this region.

Anatomical Considerations

The hip joint is a ball-in-socket joint and one of the body's largest joints. It transfers the body's weight to the lower extremities and makes upright mobility (walking and running) possible. Twenty-five muscles, including the gluteal muscles, support the hip joint around the lower pelvis. These muscles make the following actions possible: flexion, extension, abduction (extending the leg away from the midline), adduction (pulling the leg back to the midline), and internal and external rotation.

Targeting the piriformis muscles during hip mobility stretches is essential. A tight piriformis can manifest as pain in your hips, buttocks, or pelvic floor, aggravating sciatic pain. The condition can get worse during pregnancy. The piriformis stabilizes the femur in the hip joint and permits you to rotate the hip laterally and raise the thigh during hip flexion.

Hip injuries are prevalent and can include labral tears, iliopsoas impingement or snapping, bursitis, gluteus medius tears, and hip instability. Sports can often cause hip injuries. Common injuries in older adults include hip fractures, osteoarthritis (normal wear and tear of the hip joint over time), and hip dysplasia.

If you suspect that you have injured your hip(s), don't hesitate to contact your medical provider, who can administer thorough tests and examinations to correctly identify and diagnose the source of the pain and follow up with the appropriate action.

To avoid hip injuries, maintain a healthy weight and practice good posture. Incorporate resistance training, cycling, or swimming into your workouts. Sleep with a pillow between your legs. Wear comfortable, supportive shoes, and take the time to warm up and stretch before exercise. After exercise, take some time to cool down and stretch.

Instructions

Chair yoga hip exercises are a great way to strengthen your hips and improve your balance, flexibility, and range of motion. Some benefits of hip exercises include reduced risk of injury, increased mobility, improved posture, and even emotional release. You could use a yoga strap to complete any of these exercises. Use a strap, block, or pillow to modify exercise 5.

Exercise 1 – Grounding

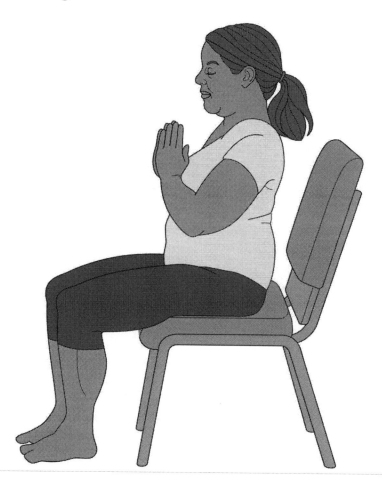

This grounding warmup invites you to connect with your body and breath to bring focus and intentionality to your practice.

Step 1: Sit up tall on your chair in a stable position. Your legs should be hip-width apart, with your knees bent at a 90-degree angle stacked above your knees. Press your feet firmly against the floor and spread your toes as wide as possible.

Step 2: Squeeze your shoulder blades together to open the front of the chest. Lower your shoulders, and nod your chin slightly toward your chest to open the back of the neck. Relax your jaw.

Step 3: Bring your hands together in a prayer position before your heart and smile.

Step 4: Close your eyes, and scan your body and mind for any tension you might be carrying.

Step 5: Take a few moments to reconnect with your breath. Consciously begin to release any tension as you exhale.

Step 6: Once you feel grounded and calm, set a simple positive intention or affirmation for your workout.

Exercise 2 – Windshield Wiper Pose

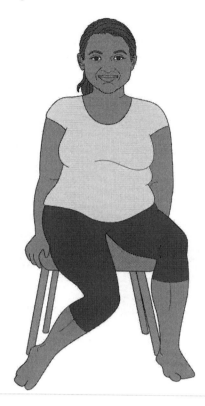

This pose promotes greater flexibility of the hip joint.

Step 1: Sit up tall on your chair.

Step 2: Gently grasp the sides of your chair and then slide your hips toward the front of your seat.

Step 3: Lean back slightly with your upper body weight supported by your arms.

Step 4: Extend your legs forward and press your heels into the floor.

Step 5: Open and close your legs repetitively like a windshield wiper, pivoting on the heels.

Step 6: Take a gentle breath in through the nose and exhale through the mouth.

Step 7: Repeat 10 to 15 times, working up to 2 reps.

Exercise 3 – Chair Pigeon Pose

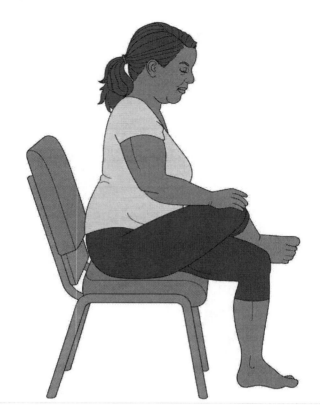

Chair pigeon pose stretches the piriformis, glutes, hip flexors, and hamstrings and opens up the hip joint.

Step 1: Sit tall in the center of your chair.

Step 2: Lift your left leg over the right as though you're going to cross your legs, but position your left calf comfortably just above the right knee.

    ✿   You can adjust this pose by crossing your left ankle over your right knee, grasping the left knee with your hands, and gently stretching it toward your body.

    ✿   You can also pull up a chair in front of you and position the left leg on that chair.

Step 3: Keep your straight back as you lower your torso toward your legs for a deeper stretch.

Step 4: Hold here for 5 to 7 deep inhalations through the nose and exhalations through the mouth.

Step 5: Repeat on the opposite side.

Exercise 4 – Seated Low Lunge

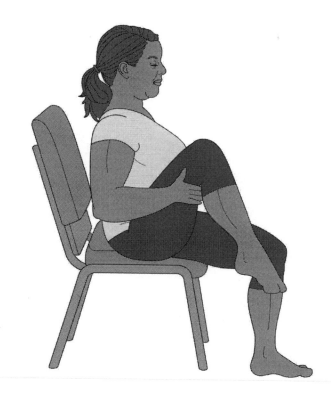

The seated low lunge opens the hamstrings and builds stability in the hips as it strengthens the pelvic floor muscles.

Step 1: Lean against the back of the chair.

Step 2: Lift your right knee to your chest.

    ✤   You can adjust the pose by looping a strap around your foot, keeping your knee bent, and lifting your leg as high as possible.

Step 3: Touch your chin to your knee.

Step 4: Hold for 5 to 7 slow breaths in the nose and out the mouth.

Step 5: Gently lower your foot to the floor and repeat on the opposite side. Work up to 2 reps.

Exercise 5 – Quadriceps Stretch

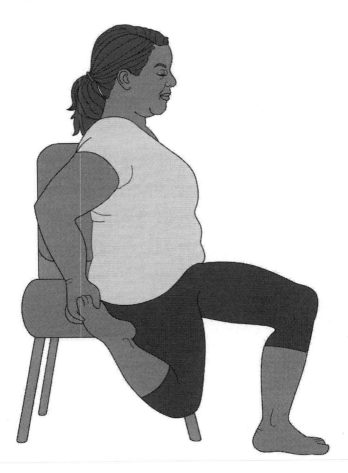

This exercise targets and stretches the hip flexors.

Step 1: Turn 90 degrees to the right in your chair and sling your right arm over the back of the chair for support. Find a stable seat, sitting tall with your right thigh and buttock fully supported. Bend your right knee at a 90-degree angle with the ankle stacked below it. Press firmly on your right foot for additional balance.

Step 2: Bend your left knee, and lift your foot toward the back of the thigh, grasping the foot with your left hand to deepen the stretch.

    ⟡   You can adjust the pose by looping a strap around your foot, lifting it as high as possible, or positioning a block or pillow under the top of your left foot.

Step 3: Hold this pose for 5 to 7 gentle breaths in through the nose and out through the mouth.

Exercise 6 – Humble Warrior

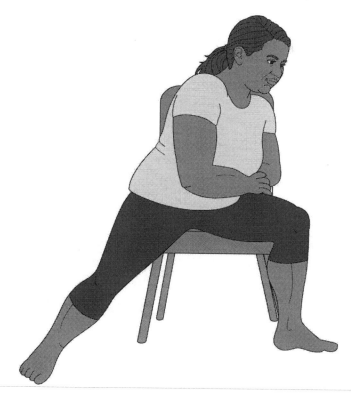

Humble warrior stretches the muscles at the front of the hips and the muscles of the inner thighs.

Step 1: Come to a comfortable and stable position near the edge of the chair.

Step 2: Open your legs wide with your knees bent and your ankles stacked below the knees.

Step 3: Keep your right knee bent at a 90-degree angle.

Step 4: Straighten your left leg, keeping your left foot flat on the floor as you position it at a 45-degree angle with your toes pointing toward your body. You'll feel this stretch on the front of your left hip.

Step 5: With a straight back, place your hands on the right thigh, and lower your chin toward your chest. You can bend your elbows and lower your torso slightly towards the thigh.

Step 6: Stay here for 5 to 7 slow breaths in through the nose and out through the mouth.

Exercise 7 – Seated Warrior Pose 1

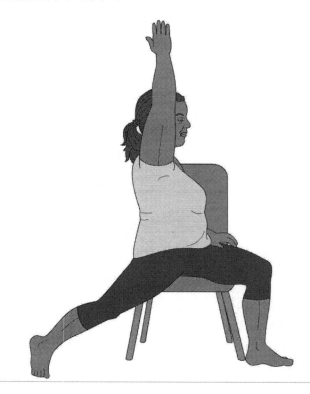

This lunge pose conditions the entire body. It specifically targets the glutes, hamstrings, hips, psoas, and quadriceps.

Step 1: Turn 90 degrees to the right in your chair. Find a stable seat, sitting tall with your right thigh and buttock fully supported. Bend your right knee at a 90-degree angle with the ankle stacked below it. Press your foot firmly on the ground for additional balance.

Step 2: Extend your left leg straight behind you. Position your foot at a 45-degree angle with the toes pointed toward your body.

Step 3: Place your right hand on your right thigh and raise your left arm to the sky. If you feel stable, lift both arms to the sky. Make sure your shoulders are relaxed, not hunched up by your ears.

Step 4: Find a point in the mid-distance and focus your gaze there.

Step 5: Stay here for 5 to 7 deep breaths in through your nose and out through your mouth.

Step 6: Repeat on the opposite side.

Exercise 8 – Wide-Legged Seated Twist

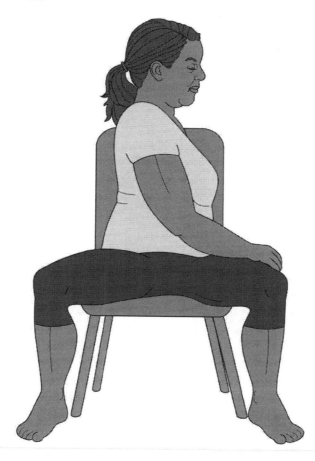

Twists are great for opening the chest and heart, and the wide-legged stance opens up the hips. Individuals with osteopenia or osteoporosis of the spine should avoid this pose.

Step 1: Find a comfortable and stable position near the edge of your chair. Open your legs wide. Gently angle your feet away from the center of your body.

Step 2: Extend your arms to either side. Bring your right hand to the opposite thigh and your left arm to the rear of the seat.

Step 3: Turn your neck to look behind you as far as possible. Focus your gaze on a point in the mid-distance.

Step 4: Hold here for 5 to 7 gentle inhalations through the nose and exhalations through the mouth.

Step 5: Repeat on the opposite side.

Exercise 9 – Integrate

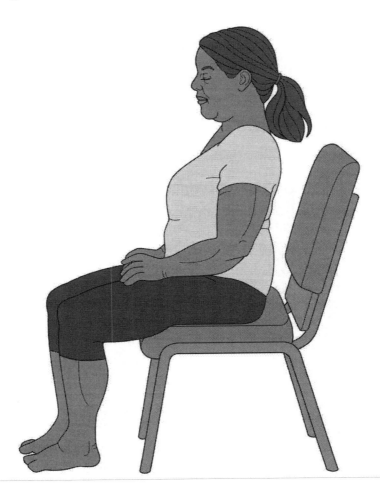

This closing exercise is an opportunity to integrate the benefits of the practice.

Step 1: Sit up tall on your chair.

Step 2: Bring your hands to rest on your thighs.

Step 3: Close your eyes, and reconnect with your breath.

Step 4: Smile gently, take a few moments to observe your feelings after the practice, and thank yourself for caring for your body and mind.

CHAPTER 11 | KNEES, ANKLES & FEET

Overview

The complexity and number of joints in your legs, from your knees to your ankles and feet, make upright mobility and various activities possible, from walking, running, jumping, and dancing to playing sports. Our lower appendages take a lot of beating, and though it's not uncommon to experience transient knee pain, it is worth investigating the underlying cause if it doesn't fade quickly.

Strong and flexible muscles support proper joint function, keeping the knees, ankles, and feet healthy and functioning over time. Injury or pain in any of these joints can prevent you from staying mobile and independent. Chair yoga is a perfect way to aid in recovery from joint replacement surgery and injuries and help you avoid future ailments.

Anatomical Considerations

The knees are the Swiss army knife of the body. They are a marvelous, multi-functional joint; no one would ever embark on a backcountry hike without them. The knee is the largest and most complex joint, designed to bear the body's weight and enable diverse types of movement. It is composed of bones, tendons, ligaments, and cartilage. The ankle is where the tibia and fibula (the lower leg bones) meet the talus (one of the foot bones). It's a joint that moves the foot in four directions. Your foot comprises 28 bones, 30 joints, and 100 muscles, ligaments, and tendons.

The knee joint is particularly vulnerable to sports and overuse injuries. The most common knee injuries include fractures, ACL injury, knee bursitis, torn meniscus, and patellar tendinitis. Compared to sports injuries, where a tumble or blunt trauma has injured the knee joint, chronic knee pain can set in with age. Wear and tear of this joint over time can give rise to knee osteoarthritis.

Ankle sprains and fractures are the most common ankle injuries, followed by tendon tears and strains. Ankle injuries can occur to people of all ages, though women over 30 have higher rates of ankle sprain than men. Injuries can occur while walking or running over uneven ground, landing poorly, tripping or falling, by blunt force in an accident, or by twisting, rolling, or rotating the ankle.

Plantar fasciitis is a common foot ailment. Symptoms include pain, stiffness, and burning in the fascia of the soles and heels of the foot. Contracted muscles, most commonly located on the arch of the foot, make walking difficult and bearing weight without intense discomfort. The feet can manifest some unpleasant but common ailments such as athlete's foot, heel spurs, hammer toes, bunions, and blisters.

Before working out, it can be beneficial to warm up and stretch your leg muscles. You can reinforce your leg joints by keeping the muscles surrounding them flexible and strong. These muscle groups include the glutes, the hamstrings and quadriceps, the inner and outer thigh muscles, the calves, and the muscles around the ankles. You can reduce your risk of ankle and foot injuries by wearing supportive footwear and ensuring that you replace your old shoes once the tread has worn down.

Instructions

In addition to building strength, leg exercises can help improve your balance and stability. This is especially important because falls are a leading cause of injury among older adults. By strengthening the muscles in your legs, you can improve your stability and reduce your risk of falling. These chair yoga exercises will help keep your knees, ankles, and feet flexible and strong. You will need a strap and a ball for this series.

Exercise 1 – Grounding

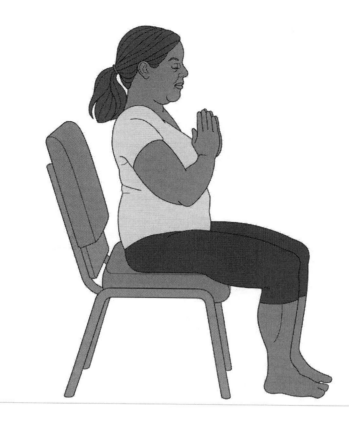

This grounding warmup invites you to connect with your body and breath to bring focus and intentionality to your practice.

Step 1: Sit up tall on your chair in a stable position. Your legs should be hip-width apart, with your knees bent at a 90-degree angle stacked above your knees. Press your feet firmly against the floor and spread your toes as wide as possible.

Step 2: Squeeze your shoulder blades together to open the front of the chest. Lower your shoulders, and nod your chin slightly toward your chest to open the back of the neck. Relax your jaw.

Step 3: Bring your hands together in a prayer position before your heart and smile.

Step 4: Close your eyes, and scan your body and mind for any tension you might be carrying.

Step 5: Take a few moments to reconnect with your breath. Consciously begin to release any tension as you exhale.

Step 6: Once you feel grounded and calm, set a simple positive intention or affirmation for your workout.

Exercise 2 – On Your Tiptoes

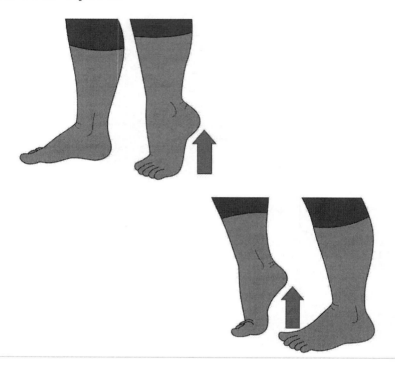

This exercise focuses on the toes, feet, and ankles. It's a beautiful stretch to warm up the lower appendages.

Step 1: Sit tall on your chair.

Step 2: Start with your feet flat on the floor. Inhale as you press your toes into the floor and lift your right heel.

Step 3: Exhale and bring your heel to the floor.

Step 4: Repeat on the opposite side.

Step 5: Do 5 to 10 heel raises on each side, working up to 2 reps.

Exercise 3 – Half Seated Forward Bend

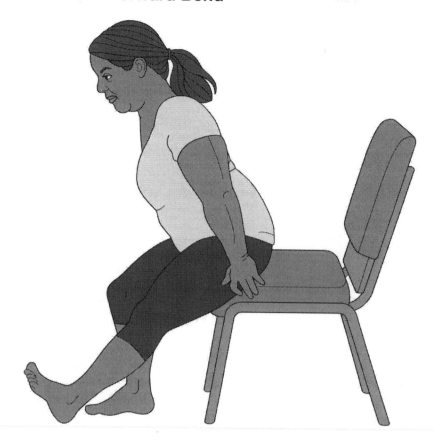

This exercise benefits the feet, ankles, hamstrings, and quadriceps.

Step 1: Scoot back on your seat.

Step 2: Hold onto the sides of the chair for balance and support.

Step 3: Extend your right leg out straight. Flex your toes slightly toward your body.

Step 4: Inhale and lengthen your spine.

Step 5: Exhale as you hinge forward from your hips and lower yourself as far as you can over your outstretched leg. You should feel a deep stretch on the back of the right leg.

Step 6: Stay here for 5 to 7 slow breaths in through the nose and out through the mouth.

Step 7: Lower your leg.

Step 8: Repeat on the opposite side. Work up to 2 reps.

Exercise 4 – Long Arc Quads

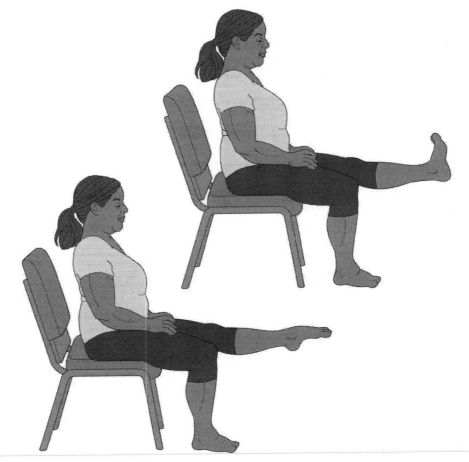

Long arc quads strengthen the quadriceps muscle, which stabilizes the knee joint.

Step 1: Sit tall on your chair.

Step 2: Lift your right leg straight in front of you with your toes pointed out.

Step 3: Engage your leg muscles by pointing your toes to your torso. Hold one full inhalation and exhalation.

Step 4: Lower your leg back to the ground.

Step 5: Repeat on the opposite leg.

Step 6: Do 10 to 15 lifts on each side, working up to 2 reps.

Exercise 5 – Foot Flex

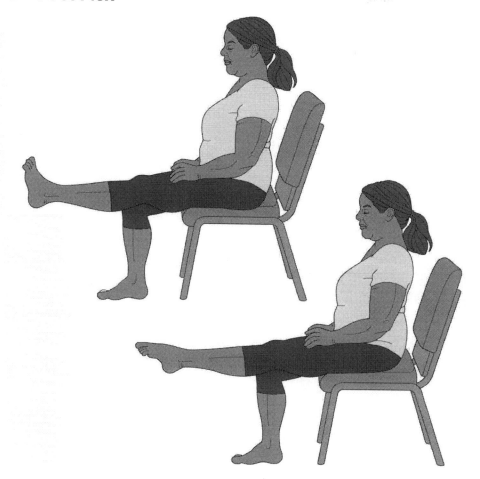

This isometric exercise strengthens the calves.

Step 1: Sit tall on your chair.

Step 2: Lift your right leg straight in front of you.

Step 3: Point your toes toward your body and hold them there for a count of ten, and then point your toes away from your body for a count of ten.

Step 4: Lower your leg back to the ground.

Step 5: Repeat on the opposite leg.

Step 6: Do 10 to 15 lifts on each side, working up to 2 reps.

Exercise 6 – Hamstring Stretch with Strap

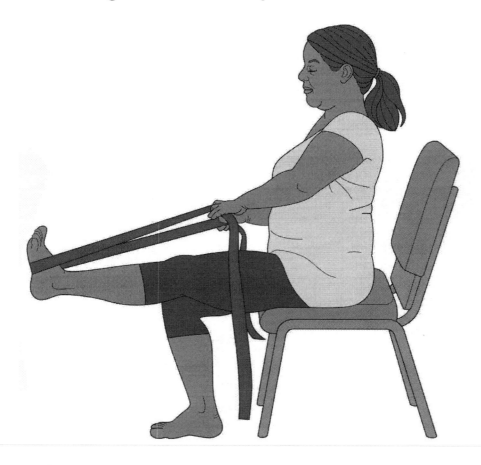

This pose stretches the hamstrings and the calf muscles, which can get tight with age and reduced activity. You'll need a strap for this pose.

Step 1: Sit tall on your chair.

Step 2: Inhale through the nose as you step your right foot into the middle of your strap or belt. Holding the strap with both hands, exhale as you straighten your right leg.

Step 3: Keep your spine elongated and adjust the intensity of the stretch by pulling the strap tighter.

Step 4: Stay here for five to seven slow breaths in through the nose and out through the mouth.

Step 5: Lower your foot to the ground and repeat on the other side.

Step 6: Work up to 2 reps.

Exercise 7 – Sit-to-Stand

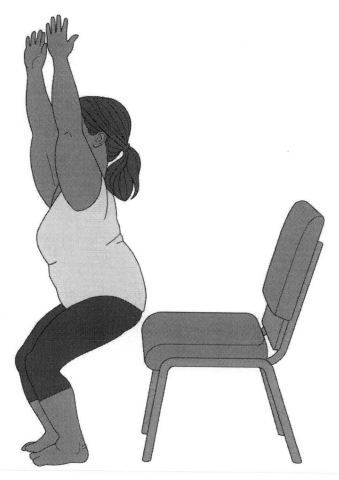

This exercise is ideal for those who have had hip or knee surgery. It strengthens core and thigh muscles and will help you transition from sitting to standing.

Step 1: Sit tall on your chair.

Step 2: Hinge forward from the hips, and squeeze your glutes and core muscles to move your center of gravity slightly forward.

Step 3: Press your feet into the ground, inhale through your nose, and stand.

Step 4: Exhale through your mouth as you carefully sit back down with slow and controlled movements.

Step 5: Repeat 5 to 10 times, working your way up to 2 reps.

Exercise 8 – Ball Exercise

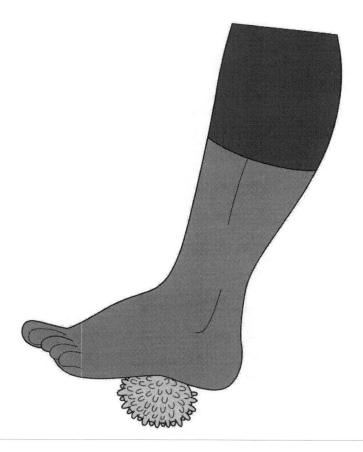

This exercise helps reduce plantar fasciitis and general foot pain.

Step 1: Sit tall on your chair.

Step 2: Inhale through the nose as you place the ball below your foot.

Step 3: Exhale through the mouth as you roll the ball toward your heels.

Step 4: Experiment with the position of the ball under your foot. Wherever you encounter a tender point, press into it to encourage the release of tension.

Step 5: Hold here for at least 5 to 7 slow breaths in through the nose and out through the mouth.

Step 6: Repeat on the opposite side.

Exercise 9 – Integrate

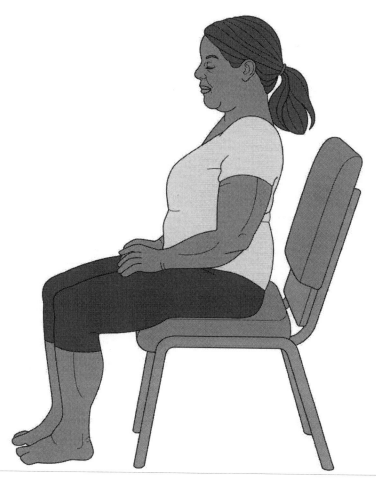

This closing exercise is an opportunity to integrate the benefits of the practice.

Step 1: Sit up tall on your chair.

Step 2: Bring your hands to rest on your thighs.

Step 3: Close your eyes, and reconnect with your breath.

Step 4: Smile gently, take a few moments to observe your feelings after the practice, and thank yourself for caring for your body and mind.

Overview

You can explore a wide range of standing poses with chair yoga. This chapter features a series of exercises that will help you improve your balance and coordination while providing a full-body workout with an extra focus on strengthening the shoulders, arms, hamstrings, ankles, and feet. The chair as a prop makes it possible to reap the benefits and gain confidence doing these poses by providing extra stability and support.

Instructions

Some exercises instruct you to focus on a fixed point on the floor or wall in the mid-distance called a drishti point, which translates from Sanskrit to English as a focal point. The drishti point will help you achieve balance in the poses, enhance your concentration, and aid you as you link your breath and body movements. Spatial data is sent from your muscles and joints to your brain, creating new neural pathways to promote long-term mobility. Practice barefoot if possible. If necessary, use a strap in exercise 3.

Please take extra precautions if you have an elevated fall risk. Practice near a wall or with an assistant. Some of these exercises include moments where you are not in contact with the chair. You can opt to replace any standing pose with a seated pose. Ease yourself slowly into any new activity. Listen intently to your body. If you begin to feel dizzy, stop immediately, and take a break until you feel normal, move to the next exercise, or stop entirely.

Exercise 1 – Grounding

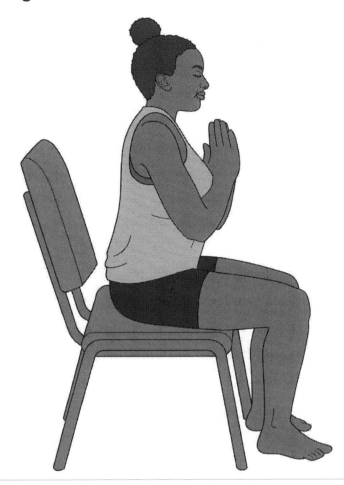

This grounding warmup invites you to connect with your body and breath to bring focus and intentionality to your practice.

Step 1: Sit up tall on your chair in a stable position. Your legs should be hip-width apart, with your knees bent at a 90-degree angle stacked above your knees. Press firmly against the floor with your feet and spread your toes as wide as possible.

Step 2: Squeeze your shoulder blades together to open the front of the chest. Lower your shoulders, and nod your chin slightly toward your chest to open the back of the neck. Relax your jaw.

Step 3: Bring your hands together in a prayer position before your heart.

Step 4: Close your eyes, and scan your body and mind for any tension you might be carrying.

Step 5: Take a few moments to reconnect with your breath. Consciously begin to release any tension as you exhale.

Step 6: Once you feel grounded and calm, set a simple positive intention or affirmation for your workout.

Exercise 2 – Heel Raises

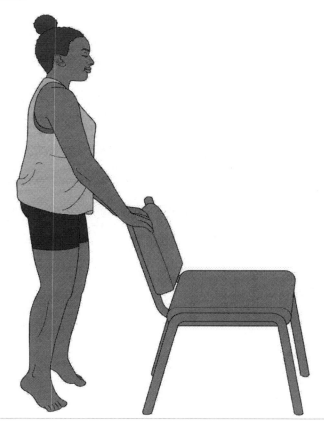

This exercise will help to strengthen the feet, ankles, and calves.

Step 1: Come to a standing position behind your chair.

Step 2: Position your legs hip-width apart with your knees gently bent. Stretch your toes as wide as you can.

Step 3: Inhale as you lift onto the balls of your feet.

Step 4: Exhale and bring your heels to the floor.

Step 5: Repeat this 5 to 10 times, working up to 2 reps.

Exercise 3 – Dancer Pose

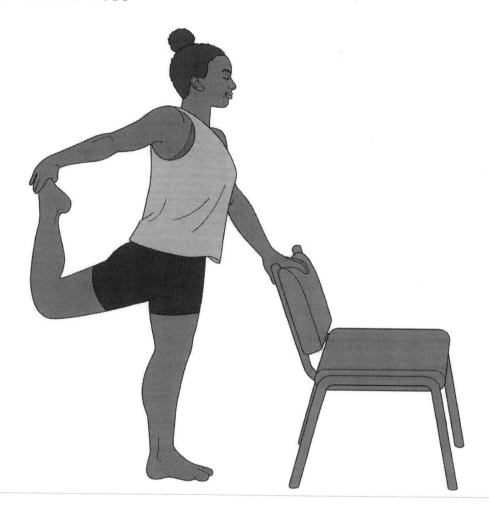

Dancer pose tones the body from head to toe as it works the arms and shoulders, biceps and triceps, chest, middle back, hips, psoas, hamstrings, feet, and ankles.

Step 1: Position yourself behind the chair about an arm's length away.

Step 2: Position your legs hip-width apart with your knees gently bent and stretch your toes as wide as possible,

Step 3: Transfer your weight to your left leg.

Step 4: Find a drishti or focus point on the floor or wall before you.

Step 5: Extend your right leg behind you. Keep your left hand on the back of the chair for support. Bend the right knee, and reach your right arm behind you to clasp your right foot.

    🌀   To adjust this pose, loop a strap around your foot and lift your foot as high as you can.

Step 6: Keep the left knee slightly bent.

Step 7: To deepen the stretch at the front of the right hip, hinge forward from the hips with a flat back as you lift your right leg higher.

Step 8: Hold here for 5 to 7 slow inhalations through the nose and exhalations through the mouth.

Step 9: Repeat on the opposite side.

Exercise 4 – Beginner Tree Pose

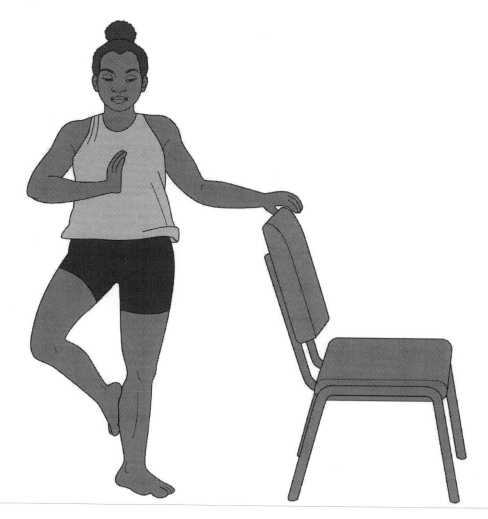

This pose is excellent for externally rotating the hips and benefits the knees, ankles, and feet.

Step 1: Come to a standing position beside your chair.

Step 2: Position your legs hip-width apart with your knees gently bent and your toes stretched wide.

Step 3: Find a drishti point on the floor or wall before you.

Step 4: Hold onto the chair with your right hand.

Step 5: Keep the toes of your left foot on the ground as you position the heel of your foot against the right inner ankle. You can also press your foot against the inner right calf. Never set the foot against the knee in this pose. Doing so can damage the knee joint.

Step 6: Swivel your left knee out at a 90-degree angle. Place your left hand on your heart.

Step 7: Stay in this position for 5 to 7 slow breaths in through the nose and out through the mouth.

Step 8: Repeat on the opposite side.

Exercise 5 – Downward-Facing Dog

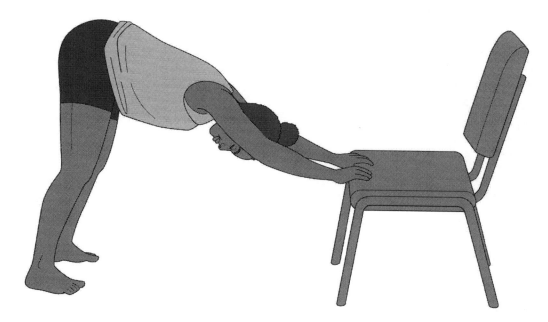

This pose benefits the arms, shoulders, lower back, gluteus muscles, and hamstrings. This pose is an inversion since the head goes below the level of the heart. Individuals with uncontrolled high blood pressure should avoid this pose.

Step 1: Stand in front of your chair, about an arm's length away.

Step 2: Position your legs hip-width apart with your knees gently bent and your toes stretched wide.

Step 3: Inhale through the nose as you raise your arms above your head.

Step 4: Exhale through the mouth as you hinge forward from your hips with a flat back. Extend your arms and rest your hands on the seat of your chair.

Step 5: Lengthen your spine and walk your heels up and down to feel the lovely stretch of the calves and hamstrings.

Step 6: Hold here for 5 to 7 deep breaths in through the nose and out through the mouth.

Step 7: To come out of the position, you can deepen the bend in your knees and hinge up from your hips, keeping your back flat with your arms raised above your head.

Step 8: Work up to 2 reps.

Exercise 6 – Standing Forward Fold

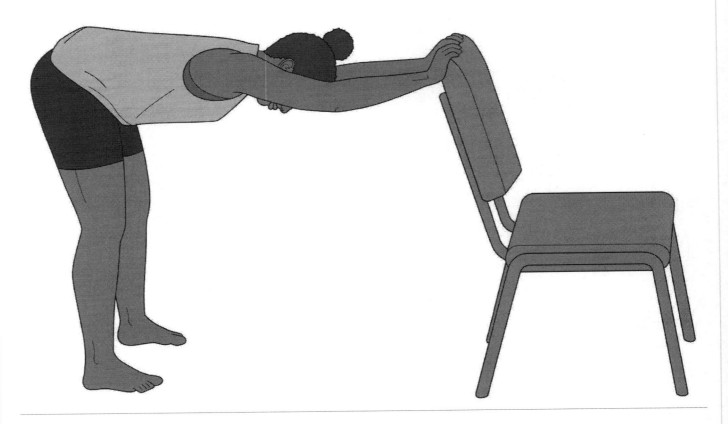

Forward fold benefits the arms, shoulders, lower back, gluteus muscles, and hamstrings.

Step 1: Position yourself behind the chair about an arm's length away.

Step 2: Position your legs hip-width apart with your knees gently bent and your toes stretched wide.

Step 3: Inhale through the nose as you raise your arms above your head.

Step 4: Exhale through the mouth as you hinge forward from your hips at a 90-degree angle. Rest your hands on the back of your chair.

Step 5: Hold here for five slow breaths in through the nose and out through the mouth.

Exercise 7 – Warrior Pose 3

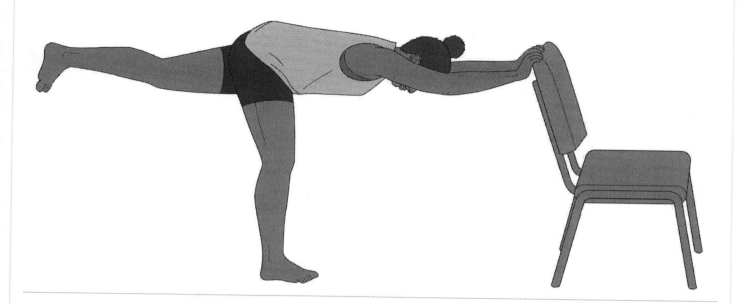

This pose stretches and strengthens the middle back, abdominals, glutes, hamstrings, pelvis, psoas, and quadriceps. It encourages internal rotation of the hips.

Step 1: Position yourself behind the chair about an arm's length away.

Step 2: Position your legs hip-width apart with your knees gently bent and your toes stretched wide.

Step 3: Inhale through the nose as you lift your arms above your head and exhale through your mouth as you hinge forward from your hips with a flat back to a 90-degree angle.

Step 4: Rest your hands on the back of the chair.

Step 5: Lift your right leg behind you as high as possible, keeping your hips level.

Step 6: Hold here for 5 to 7 slow breaths in through the nose and out through the mouth.

Step 7: To come out of this position, lower your right leg to the floor, bend your knees, and hinge up from the hips with a flat back to a standing position.

Step 8: Repeat on the opposite side.

Exercise 8 – Warrior Pose 1

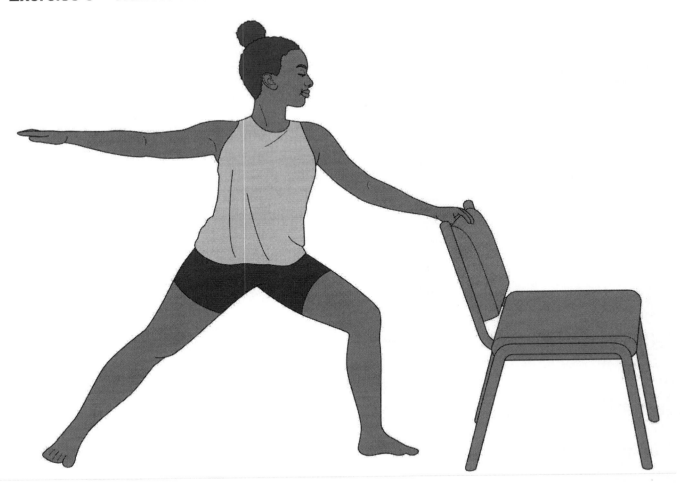

This variation of the warrior pose benefits the whole body. It targets the feet, knees, ankles, hamstrings, hips, and pelvis. It promotes external rotation of the hips.

Step 1: Position yourself behind the chair about an arm's length away.

Step 2: Position your legs hip-width apart with your knees gently bent and your toes stretched wide.

Step 3: Extend your left leg behind you, and angle your left foot at a 45-degree angle with your toes pointing forward.

Step 4: Bend your right knee, coming into a lunge. Ensure that you keep your right knee stacked above your ankle so that you can see your front right toe. Take care not to collapse the knee inward.

Step 5: Inhale through the nose as you lift your arms above your head. Drop your right hand to the top of the chair, and extend your left arm behind you.

Step 6: Find a drishti point on the wall before you.

Step 7: Hold this pose for 5 to 7 slow breaths in through the nose and out through the mouth.

Step 8: To come out of the pose, slowly slide your left leg forward as you straighten your right leg and lower your left arm.

Step 9: Repeat on the opposite side.

Exercise 9 – Integrate

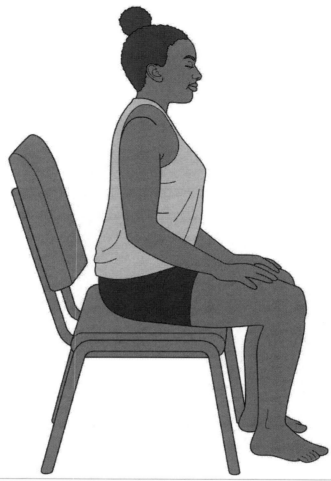

This closing exercise is an opportunity to integrate the benefits of the practice.

Step 1: Sit up tall on your chair.

Step 2: Bring your hands to rest on your thighs.

Step 3: Close your eyes, and reconnect with your breath.

Step 4: Smile gently, take a few moments to observe your feelings after the practice, and thank yourself for caring for your body and mind.

CHAPTER 13 | FULL-BODY 10-MINUTE WORKOUT

Overview

This selection of chair yoga exercises is fantastic for anyone seeking a full-body workout that you can easily integrate into your daily routine at home or in the office. The length of the practice depends on how long you spend on each exercise and whether you do repetitions or not, so you can adjust it according to your needs. You can create your own full-body chair yoga routine by mixing and matching exercises from each chapter to target specific muscle groups.

Instructions

This full-body routine includes a mix of sitting and standing postures. If you do not feel comfortable with the standing exercises, feel free to substitute seated exercises from another chapter. In the fourth exercise, you can use blocks under your hands to modify the forward fold.

Exercise 1 – Grounding

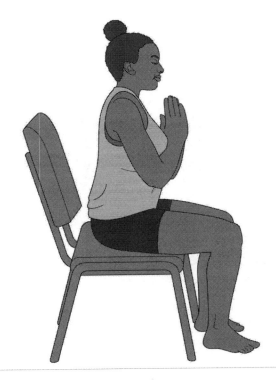

This grounding warmup invites you to connect with your body and breath to bring focus and intentionality to your practice.

Step 1: Sit up tall on your chair in a stable position. Your legs should be hip-width apart, with your knees bent at a 90-degree angle stacked above your knees. Press firmly against the floor with your feet and spread your toes as wide as possible.

Step 2: Squeeze your shoulder blades together to open the front of the chest. Lower your shoulders, and nod your chin slightly toward your chest to open the back of the neck. Relax your jaw.

Step 3: Bring your hands together in a prayer position before your heart.

Step 4: Close your eyes, and scan your body and mind for any tension you might be carrying.

Step 5: Take a few moments to reconnect with your breath. Consciously begin to release any tension as you exhale.

Step 6: Once you feel grounded and calm, set a simple positive intention or affirmation for your workout.

Exercise 2 – Neck "V" Rotation

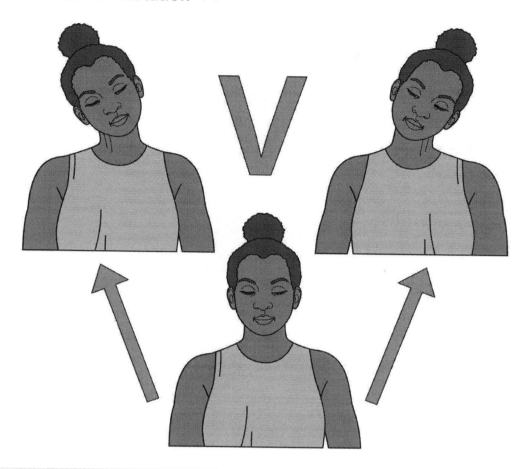

This exercise is excellent for releasing muscle tension at the back of the neck.

Step 1: Sit tall on your chair.

Step 2: Imagine that you will be tracing a "V" shape with your chin.

Step 3: Inhale through the nose as you lift your chin to the upper left. Exhale through the mouth as you lower your chin to the top of your chest.

Step 4: Inhale through the nose as you lift your chin to the upper right. Exhale through the mouth as you lower your chin to the top of your chest.

Step 5: Repeat this 10 to 15 times on each side.

Exercise 3 – Seated Twist

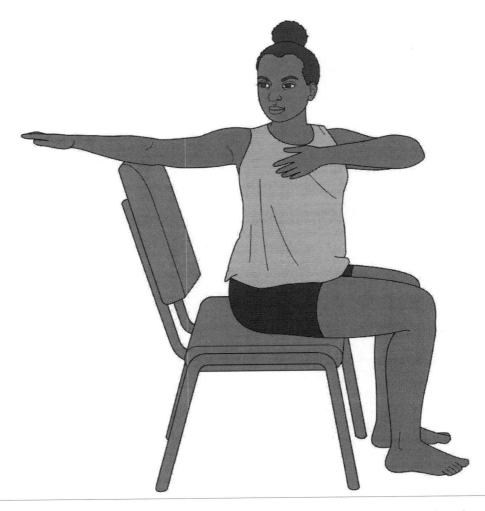

The seated twist benefits the neck, the upper and middle back, and the chest. Individuals with osteopenia or osteoporosis of the spine should avoid this pose.

Step 1: Sit tall on your chair.

Step 2: Inhale through the nose and extend both arms before you.

Step 3: Exhale through the mouth as you twist to the left. Your left arm will point backward. Turn your neck and gaze behind you. Bring your right palm to rest on your chest.

Step 4: Hold here for 5 to 7 gentle breaths in through the nose and out through the mouth.

Step 5: Repeat on the opposite side, working up to 2 reps.

Exercise 4 – Seated Forward Fold

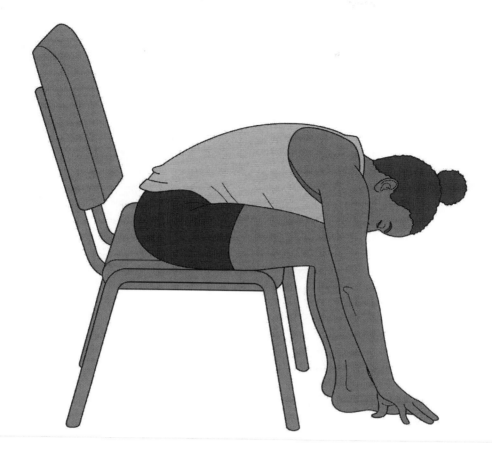

This exercise brings relief to the lower back and glutes. This pose is an inversion since the head goes below the level of the heart. There are modifications offered for those who have untreated high blood pressure.

Step 1: Sit tall on your chair.

Step 2: Inhale through the nose. As you exhale, hinge forward from your hips as you lower your torso toward your thighs.

Step 3: Bring your hands to the floor and drop your head between your knees.
- 🌀 To adjust this pose, place blocks below your hands or lower your torso slightly and support yourself with your hands on your thighs.

Step 4: Stay here for 5 to 7 gentle breaths through the nose and out through the mouth.

Step 5: Return to the sitting position and repeat on the other side, working up to 2 reps.

Exercise 5 – Standing Side Bend

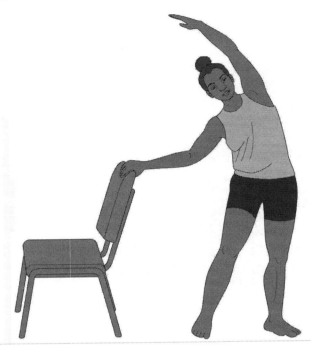

Standing side bend stretches the lateral body, encouraging good posture and deep breathing by opening the intercostal muscles and lengthening the lower back muscles.

Step 1: Stand behind your chair.

Step 2: Relax your jaw, elongate your spine, and squeeze your shoulder blades together. Relax the tops of your shoulders downward, and gently nod your chin toward your chest. Position your legs hip-width apart with your knees gently bent. Stretch your toes wide.

Step 3: Hold the back of the chair with your right arm for support.

Step 4: Lift your left arm above your head.

Step 5: Shift your weight to your left hip and gently bend your torso and arm to the right. Be careful not to collapse your chest here. Keep your core stable by squeezing your lower abdominal muscles.

Step 6: Hold this pose for 5 to 7 slow breaths in through the nose and out through the mouth.

Step 7: Repeat on the opposite side.

Exercise 6 – One-Legged Heel Raises

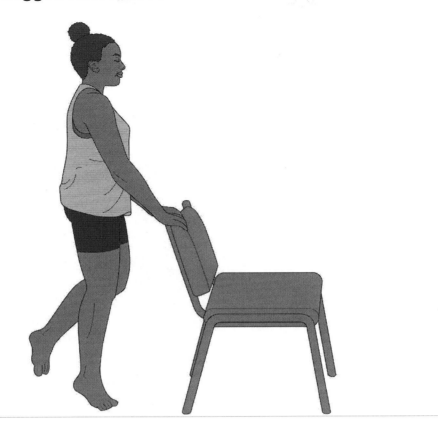

One-legged heel raises encourage good balance and are great for the feet, ankles, and calves.

Step 1: Come to a standing position behind your chair.

Step 2: Elongate your spine, and squeeze your shoulder blades together. Relax the tops of your shoulders downward, and gently nod your chin toward your chest. Position your legs hip-width apart with your knees gently bent. Stretch your toes as wide as you can, and increase the surface area of your feet as they touch the floor.

Step 3: Lift onto the ball of your right foot if comfortable, or stand flat on the floor.

Step 4: Bend your left knee as you lift your left foot to a 90-degree angle.

Step 5: Lower both feet back to the floor. Repeat 10 to 15 times, working up to 2 reps.

Step 6: Repeat on the opposite side.

Exercise 7 – Half Forward Fold

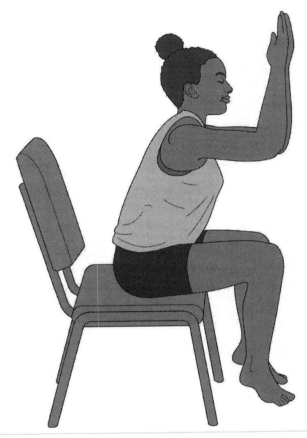

This exercise is ideal for the arms, shoulders, feet, ankles, hips, and psoas muscles.

Step 1: Sit tall on your chair.

Step 2: Lift your heels and balance your weight on the balls of your feet. Hinge your torso slightly forward from the hips. Lift your arms straight before you, bend your elbows at a 90-degree angle, and press your forearms and hands together.

Step 3: Stay here for 5 to 7 slow breaths in through the nose and out through the mouth, working up to 2 reps.

Exercise 8 – Pigeon Pose with Raised Arms

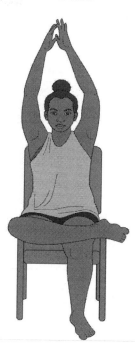

This exercise strengthens the shoulders and relieves sore glutes, hips, hamstrings, feet, and ankles.

Step 1: Sit tall on your chair.

Step 2: Lift your left leg over the right as though you're going to cross your legs, but position your lower leg (just above the ankle) comfortably on the right thigh (just above the knee).

- ⟳ Alternatively, lift your left leg as though crossing it over the right, but instead of positioning your lower leg on the right thigh, grasp your knee with your hands and gently stretch it to the right to decrease pressure on the knee joint. Skip the next step.

Step 3: Inhale your arms above your head, pressing the palms of your hands together.

Step 4: To deepen the pose, keep a straight back as you lower your torso towards your legs.

Step 5: Hold here for 5 to 7 deep inhalations through the nose and exhalations through the mouth.

Step 6: Repeat on the opposite side.

Exercise 9 – Integrate

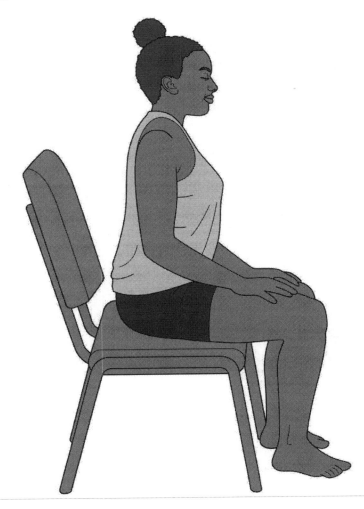

This closing exercise is an opportunity to integrate the benefits of the practice.

Step 1: Sit up tall on your chair.

Step 2: Bring your hands to rest on your thighs.

Step 3: Close your eyes, and reconnect with your breath.

Step 4: Smile gently, take a few moments to observe your feelings after the practice, and thank yourself for caring for your body and mind.

Overview

This routine features a variety of chair yoga exercises that target the body from head to toe. Your body will thank you for the extra time and attention you devote to it! Adjust it according to your needs; the length of any routine depends on how long you stay in each posture and whether you add repetitions. This flow is ideal for anyone seeking a comprehensive workout.

Instructions

Find a convenient time to devote yourself to this full-body 20-minute routine. You will feel more flexible, relaxed, and confident. It consists of a mix of sitting and standing postures. You can create a customized full-body routine by mixing and matching your favorite exercises. Use this routine as a template. You can use a strap or blocks to adjust the poses if needed.

Exercise 1 – Grounding

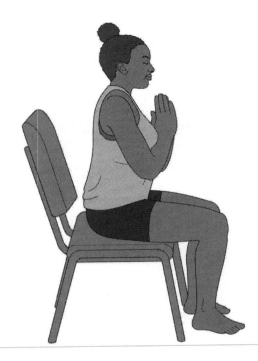

This grounding warmup invites you to connect with your body and breath to bring focus and intentionality to your practice.

Step 1: Sit up tall on your chair in a stable position. Your legs should be hip-width apart, with your knees bent at a 90-degree angle stacked above your knees. Press firmly against the floor with your feet and spread your toes as wide as possible.

Step 2: Squeeze your shoulder blades together to open the front of the chest. Lower your shoulders, and nod your chin slightly toward your chest to open the back of the neck. Relax your jaw.

Step 3: Bring your hands together in a prayer position before your heart.

Step 4: Close your eyes, and scan your body and mind for any tension you might be carrying.

Step 5: Take a few moments to reconnect with your breath. Consciously begin to release any tension as you exhale.

Step 6: Once you feel grounded and calm, set a simple positive intention or affirmation for your workout.

Exercise 2 – Upper Arm Stretch

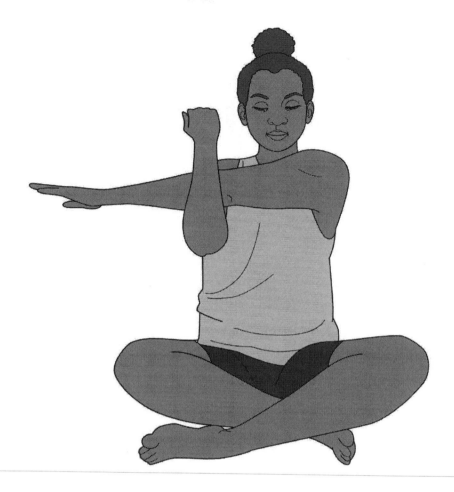

This exercise stretches the deltoids, which keep the shoulder joint strong.

Step 1: Sit tall on your chair.

Step 2: Cross your left arm across your chest. Press it with the right hand above the elbow joint.

Step 3: Inhale slowly through the nose and exhale through the mouth for 5 to 7 breaths.

Step 4: Repeat on the opposite side.

Step 5: Work up to 2 reps.

Exercise 3 – Overhead Shoulder Stretch

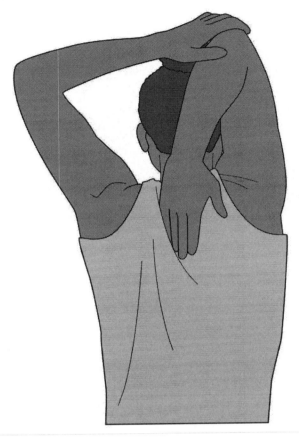

This exercise increases shoulder mobility and flexibility.

Step 1: Sit tall on your chair.

Step 2: Lift your left arm straight up, bend your elbow, and rest your palm on the back of your head, neck, or upper back.

Step 3: Grasp your left elbow with the right hand. Bend to the right to deepen the stretch.

Step 4: Inhale slowly through the nose and exhale through the mouth for 5 to 7 breaths.

Step 5: Repeat on the opposite side.

Exercise 4 – Hands Up

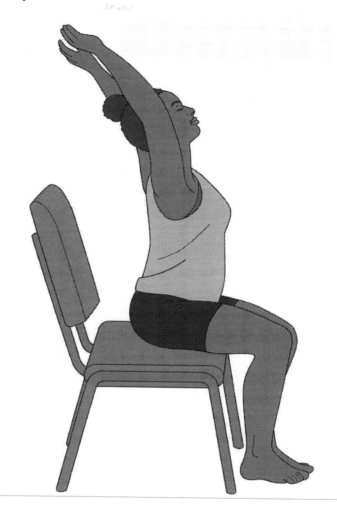

Hands up targets the arms, shoulders, and chest.

Step 1: Sit tall on your chair.

Step 2: Raise your arms above your head, lifting your chin to the sky and arching your back slightly as you open your chest.

　🌀　Alternatively, keep your elbows bent and raise them as high as you can, or lift just one arm at a time.

Step 3: Inhale slowly through the nose and exhale through the mouth for 5 to 7 breaths.

Step 4: Work up to 2 reps.

Exercise 5 – Side Bend Eagle Pose

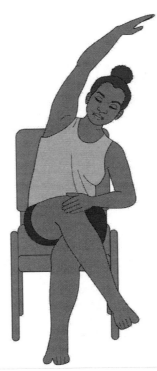

This exercise stretches the middle and upper back and targets the glutes, hips, and legs.

Step 1: Sit tall on your chair.

Step 2: Cross your left leg over your right leg. Grasp your left thigh with the right hand.

Step 3: Lift your left arm above your head and gently stretch your torso to the right side. Make sure not to collapse your chest inwards.

Step 4: Keep your right foot pressed into the ground and your left hip anchored to the chair seat.

Step 5: Inhale slowly through the nose and exhale through the mouth for 5 to 7 breaths.

Step 6: Repeat on the opposite side.

Step 7: Work up to 2 reps.

Exercise 6 – Eagle Pose

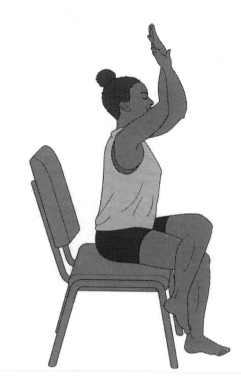

The eagle pose benefits the arms, shoulders, upper back, and knees.

Step 1: Sit tall on your chair.

Step 2: Cross your left leg over the right leg at the knee. If you can't cross your leg over the knee, you can cross your shins or ankles.

Step 3: Extend your arms straight out on either side of you. Bend your elbows at a 90-degree angle. Cross your right arm under your left and hug yourself.

Step 4: Press the backs of your forearms together, and lift your arms to the sky. Stay in the hug position if this isn't comfortable.

Step 5: Stay here for 5 to 7 slow breaths in through the nose and out through the mouth.

Step 6: Repeat on the opposite side.

Step 7: Work up to 2 reps.

Exercise 7 – Head-to-Knee

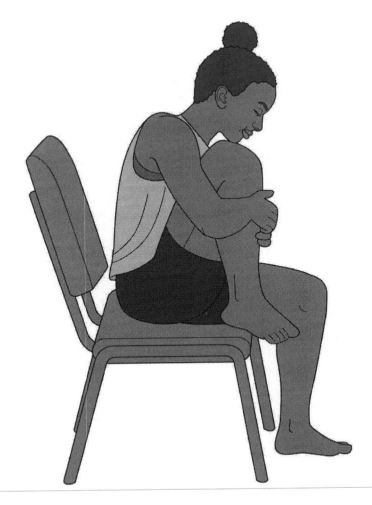

This exercise will target your hips, glutes, and knees.

Step 1: Sit tall on your chair.

Step 2: Lift your right knee to your chest, resting your foot on the chair seat. Drop your forehead to the knee.

Step 3: Inhale slowly through the nose and exhale through the mouth for 5 to 7 breaths.

Step 4: Repeat on the opposite side.

Step 5: Work up to 2 reps.

Exercise 8 – Standing Twist

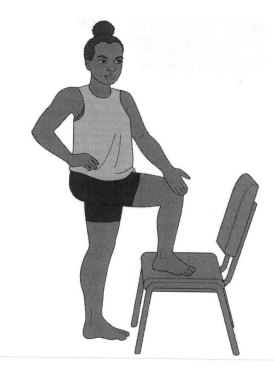

Standing twist targets the lower back, the hips, internal rotation of the hips, and the psoas muscles. Those with osteopenia or osteoporosis of the spine should avoid this pose.

Step 1: Stand facing the front of your chair, about an arm's length away.

Step 2: Position your legs hip-width apart with your knees gently bent and your toes stretched wide.

Step 3: Lift your left leg onto the center of the chair or a block.

Step 4: Place the back of your left hand on the thigh just behind your knee joint.

Step 5: Place your right hand on your right hip and gently twist to the right. Look over your right shoulder.

Step 6: Inhale slowly through the nose and exhale through the mouth for 5 to 7 breaths.

Step 7: Repeat on the opposite side.

Step 8: Work up to 2 reps.

Exercise 9 – Standing Quad Stretch

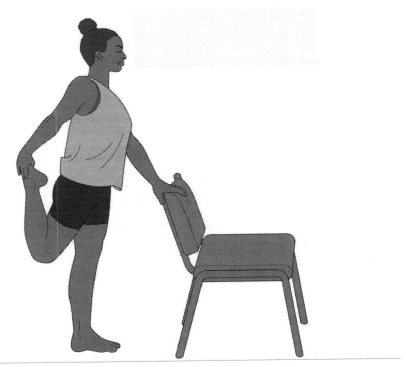

The standing quad stretch is excellent for feet, ankles, hamstrings, knees, and quadriceps.

Step 1: Stand behind your chair, about an arm's length away.

Step 2: Position your legs hip-width apart with your knees gently bent and your toes stretched wide.

Step 3: Lift your left heel to the back of your thigh or as high as possible, and grasp the left foot with your left hand.

    ✿   You can adjust this pose by looping the strap around your foot. Or take a step backward with your left foot and then shift your weight through the front of the left hip to open up the hip flexors.

Step 4: Inhale slowly through the nose and exhale through the mouth for 5 to 7 breaths.

Step 5: Repeat on the opposite side.

Step 6: Work up to 2 reps.

Exercise 10 – Triangle Pose

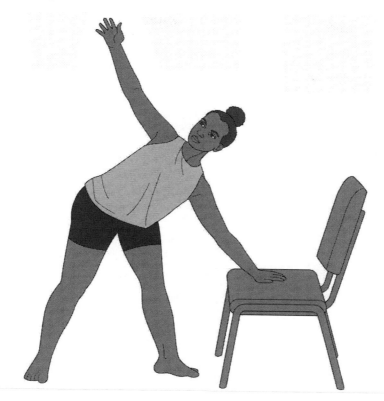

The triangle pose engages the whole body and increases core muscle strength.

Step 1: Stand facing the front of your chair, about a step away.

Step 2: Position your legs hip-width apart with your knees gently bent and your toes stretched wide.

Step 3: Widen your stance by stepping your right foot back and positioning it at a 90-degree angle. Your left foot will face the chair.

Step 4: Extend your arms out to either side. Shift forward and place your left hand on the seat of the chair. You can rest your right hand on your hip or reach toward the sky. You can direct your gaze to the sky, straight forward, or at the floor.

Step 5: Inhale slowly through the nose and exhale through the mouth for 5 to 7 breaths.

Step 6: Repeat on the opposite side.

Step 7: Work up to 2 reps.

Exercise 11 – Forward Bend

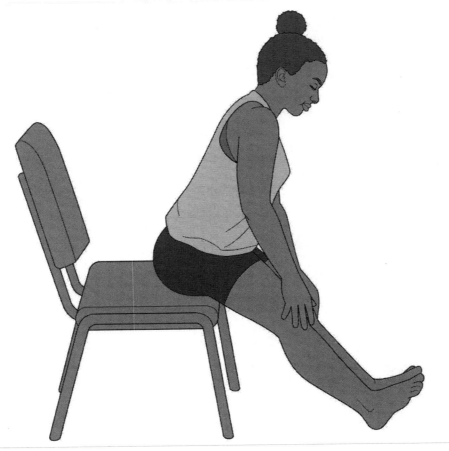

Forward bend opens up the hamstrings and the lower back.

Step 1: Sit tall near the edge of your chair.

Step 2: Extend your legs in front of you.

Step 3: Press your heels into the floor with your toes pointing up.

Step 4: Extend your arms as you hinge forward from the hips, keeping your back straight. Once you feel the stretch, lower your hands to your thighs, close your eyes, and focus on your breath.

Step 5: Inhale slowly through the nose and exhale through the mouth for 5 to 7 breaths.

Step 6: Repeat on the opposite side.

Step 7: Work up to 2 reps.

Exercise 12 – Integrate

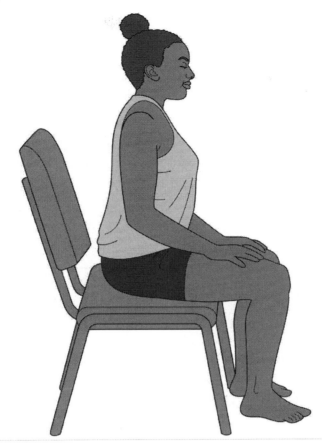

This closing exercise is an opportunity to integrate the benefits of the practice.

Step 1: Sit up tall on your chair.

Step 2: Bring your hands to rest on your thighs.

Step 3: Close your eyes, and reconnect with your breath.

Step 4: Smile gently, take a few moments to observe your feelings after the practice, and thank yourself for caring for your body and mind.

C H A P T E R 15 | MEDITATION

Overview

The mind is a master in creating mental chaos. Its ability to whip a simple thought into a completely unrelated drama is unprecedented. One moment, you're thinking about what kind of pizza to pick up for dinner, and the next, you're reliving a conflict you had with your boss ten years ago, which triggers an emotional reaction and a cascade of stress hormones. "But wait," you realize, red in the face, "wasn't I trying to decide between a 4-cheese pizza or a margarita pizza?" Mindfulness, a meditation technique, gives you the tools to name, observe and release such an experience rather than stumbling deeper into the spiral.

What comes before thought if thoughts create words, words create actions, and actions create reality? Meditation is the best open-ended exploration of that question, and the quest begins by simply observing the mind, the body, the senses, and each passing moment. Some might call the space before thought divinity or higher spiritual consciousness; others might call it stillness and calm.

Cultivating meditative practice can support your physical and mental health and lay the groundwork for profound shifts in how you relate to the world. The key is to do so without judgment and with an open heart. Doing so makes it possible to notice patterns by creating space between thoughts and distancing yourself from identifying with them.

Meditation became a refuge for me after getting divorced. I started attending silent meditation retreats. When you lose everything that once defined who you were, a complex tapestry of identity unravels, and you find yourself holding the strands of the present in your hands, at a complete loss for what the future might hold. Sitting quietly and befriending your heart amid staggering loss is a good place to start.

Roots of Meditation

The word meditation in English comes from the mid-16th century Latin root word meditat (contemplation). Archaeological evidence of meditative practices has been unearthed in Egypt, the Indus Valley of Pakistan, and China. In ancient Eastern traditions, some five thousand years BC, religions emerged from the profound act of stilling the mind.

Meditation spread via the Silk Road and is the loom upon which Buddhism, Jainism, Hinduism, and Sikhism are woven. Meditation practices also infused Judaism and Islam. Early Christianity incorporated different meditation practices in the East and West: hesychasm and Lectio Divina. Prayer, scripture, and contemplation were vital components.

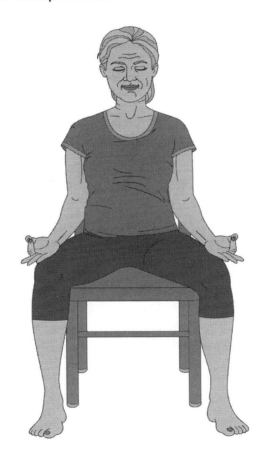

Mudras

You might have encountered mudras while taking a yoga class or looking at religious art. You would have seen your teacher or a religious figure with their fingers and hands positioned in a specific way. Each position has a meaning behind it. Mudra, which translates to seal, is a hand gesture that embodies an intention. You can experiment with the various mudra during your chair yoga meditation practice.

Anjali (offering) mudra – This mudra is called the "prayer position." In this position, bring your palms together, leaving a small space between the palms and the fingers to represent the heart's opening.

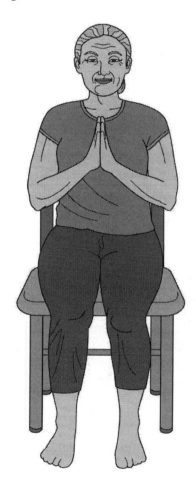

Gyan (wisdom) mudra – This is a common mudra representing knowledge. Create a little circle by bringing your thumb and forefinger together. It can enhance concentration and stability during meditation.

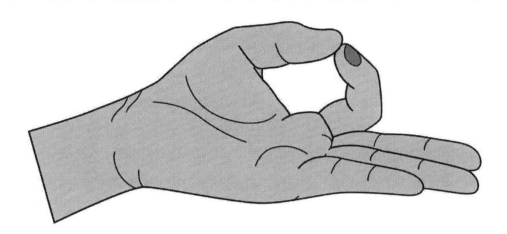

Dhyana (perception) mudra – This mudra calms the meditator and encourages depth of awareness. Cradle the right hand in the left hand and bring the tips of the thumbs together.

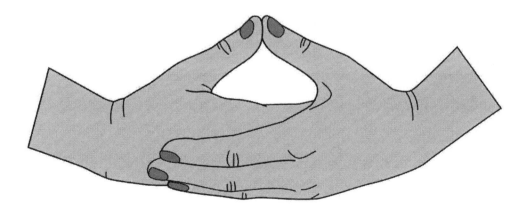

Garuda Mudra – This mudra represents an eagle, the king of birds, and is thought to enhance the qualities of inner freedom and vitality within the meditator. With your palms facing your body, bring the pads of your thumbs together to touch. Bring the hands to rest in the center of the chest.

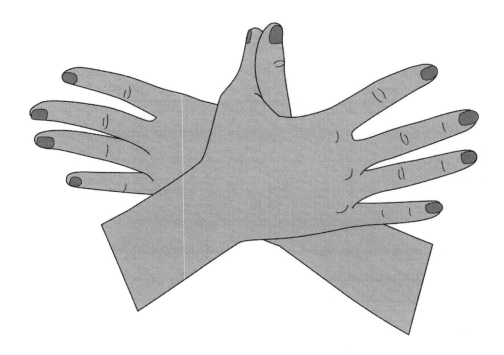

Anatomical Considerations

Research indicates that people with anxiety, asthma, cancer, chronic pain, depression, post-traumatic stress disorder (PTSD), heart disease, high blood pressure, irritable bowel syndrome (IBS), and tension headaches may benefit from regular meditation practice.

Meditation can also:

- Help you sleep better
- Boost positive emotions
- Increase self-awareness and presence
- Increase creativity and patience
- Strengthen the ability to take new perspectives in stressful situations
- Lower resting heart rate and blood pressure levels

Did you know that the brain produces electromagnetic waves that change in frequency and intensity according to the activity it is engaged in? Brain cells generate electricity to communicate with each other, radiating this information through brain waves measurable with an electroencephalogram (EEG) monitor.

Delta waves – (0.5 to 3) hertz are the slowest and most profound of the brainwaves. Delta waves are created during deep, dreamless sleep when the body is engaged in healing and regeneration.

Theta waves – (3 to 8 hertz) occur while dreaming, falling asleep, waking up, and during deep meditation. This frequency corresponds with vivid imagery, intuition, and memory.

Alpha waves – (8 to 12 hertz) are created when the brain is at ease in the present moment and can arise during some meditative states. Alpha waves occur during states of alertness and mind and body coordination.

Beta waves – (12 to 38 hertz) are generated while interacting with the outside world and cognitive tasks. Beta waves are further divided into three bands corresponding to the intensity of the activity at hand. They increase during intense problem-solving, excitement or stimulation, and anxiety. High-frequency processing can be exhausting for the brain as beta waves require a lot of energy to produce.

Gamma waves – (38 to 42 hertz) are the fastest and most subtle waves that conduct information in a quiet and expedited manner. They occur during moments of happiness, and their presence indicates excellent memory and high IQ levels.

You can train your brain to slow its brainwaves into meditative alpha and theta states through yoga, pranayama, and meditation. Brainwave awareness can help you optimize your routine. In the morning, for example, the last thing you want to do is scroll on your phone. Just after waking, your intensely creative theta brainwaves are flowing, and you can use that time to recall your dreams, visualize your goals, and journal. Meditation practice just before bed can work wonders for those with sleep problems because it can slow overactive beta waves whipped up during the day.

Studies indicate meditation activates the "rest and digest" response of the parasympathetic nervous system, which slows heart and breath rate, relaxes muscles, increases blood flow throughout the body, optimizes digestion, and counteracts the effects of stress and anxiety on your body.

Long-term meditation increases the density of gray matter in the hippocampus and frontal regions of the brain, optimizing cognition and memory, which results in better fact retention and mindful behavior. It also increases anterior insula and cortical thickness, which is linked to high levels of self-awareness and increased attention span. In short, you'll keep your mind sharp and focused if you meditate!

Types of Meditation

Guided Meditation and Yoga Nidra – Guided meditation is a beautiful practice for beginners that takes the "So I'm sitting on a cushion to meditate, now what?" guesswork out of the process. It consists of following a person's voice as they guide you through a meditation that uses the power of visualization to relax your body and tap into your slower brain waves. You might journey through the senses, walk along an empty beach, or do a body scan. Following the cues and feeling the benefits during and after practicing will help you gain confidence in meditating.

You might have seen advertisements for Yoga Nidra classes and wondered what they are; translated from Sanskrit, it means yogic sleep. It is a practice that involves setting an intention to focus on your deepest desire at the beginning of a guided meditation, such as "I am happy and healthy," "I am strong and independent," or "love." This practice helps participants tap into deep inner peace and relaxation while cultivating positive intentions.

Zen and Mindfulness Meditation – Zen meditation is an ancient Buddhist practice described as not-thinking, the art of sitting completely still while keeping the eyes slightly open. Zen meditation focuses on cultivating a universal state of consciousness.

Mindfulness meditation arose from Zen meditation, yet it is a secular practice that anyone from any religion can practice. The goal is to bring non-judgmental awareness to each moment to reduce habitual reactivity. Through this practice, you'll strengthen your observation skills by learning to label your experiences. You'll begin to recognize thoughts, emotions, and sensations for what they are without assigning additional significance to them.

You can practice mindfulness anytime when you bring your full attention to the present moment. You can do it while drinking tea, washing the dishes, or even commuting to work. Try setting your phone aside while eating a meal and savoring the flavors of every bite. The intention is to let the experiences pass through you and release them without clinging to them. Spending time in nature and simply observing your surroundings is a great way to deepen your mindfulness practice.

Mantra and Japa meditation – Mantra meditation involves repeating a sound, word, or phrase. It can be spoken aloud, sung, whispered, or silently repeated while seated with eyes closed. The beauty of mantra meditation is that you actively guide your mind during the practice, and it is possible to find deep relaxation and calm.

It is a beautiful way to shift one's mindset from rumination or worry to a more positive track. When I am anxious or feel lonely, I repeat a comforting mantra during these moments. It might even be when I'm on an airplane, hiking, or in a group of unfamiliar people; it is a touchstone that calms my mind.

The power of repetition of a sacred word or prayer is a nearly universal concept across religions. The use of prayer beads while repeating a mantra is called Japa meditation in Jainism, Sikhism, Buddhism, and Hinduism. In Catholicism, prayers are made using the rosary. The sensory experience of connecting mantras to prayer beads can guide you into deep contemplation.

Loving-Kindness Meditation or Metta Meditation – Loving-kindness meditation is about receiving and sending unconditional love to yourself and others. It follows a sequence of visualizing joy, happiness, or the image of someone in your life who had your best interests at heart and whose love positively touched your life. The meditation asks you to open your heart to receive their love and to invite yourself to feel worthy of it. The practice then extends to sending these feelings of joy, happiness, and love to those you care for. More advanced versions of the method include sending this love to those with whom you have conflicts and strangers.

Vipassana and Hridaya Meditation – Vipassana meditation, which means seeing things as they are in Sanskrit, is an ancient practice to free oneself from suffering. It's a 10-day silent meditation course offered free worldwide. The technique is simple but requires great discipline. Participants focus on the breath as it enters in and out of the nose and continuously return there when they realize the mind has strayed.

Hridaya meditation, which translates to spiritual heart meditation, invites participants to focus on the heart as the seat of the soul. This tradition draws upon wisdom from across all religious traditions. They offer relatively affordable silent retreats, allowing participants to dive deep into their practice.

Instructions

If you are currently undergoing psychological treatment – Please consult your psychologist before trying these techniques. Do not use these exercises to replace professional psychological advice, diagnosis, or treatment.

Please seek professional support – Meditation can sometimes evoke unpleasant experiences such as emotional discomfort, agitation, or anxiety. These feelings are a natural part of connecting with the full spectrum of your emotions. Nevertheless, please seek additional psychological support if they feel unmanageable or overwhelming for you.

You can meditate anytime, anywhere. Like any new activity, it can take time to create a habit, so challenge yourself to make time and space in your daily routine to start a technique that appeals to you and stick with it for at least two weeks! Start with small, achievable goals, like five minutes daily, and celebrate when you accomplish them.

Create a special place for your chair yoga, pranayama, and meditation practice. Use a diffuser with your favorite essential oil, burn a stick of incense, or light a candle to create a reverent mood. You can use a weighted eye pillow while lying down, an eye mask while seated, and earplugs to block distractions if these options appeal to you. If you like to meditate to music, find a great playlist, and don't hesitate to get a comfortable meditation cushion for your chair.

In these meditations, follow the natural rhythm of your breath. There is no need to shift your breathing rate faster or slower. If possible, breathe in through your nose and out through your mouth.

It's not necessary to sit on the floor cross-legged to meditate! You can do all the following exercises sitting on your chair or lying down. If you lie down, do so with palms facing up and feet hip-width apart. Use a thin pillow behind your head if you need support.

Exercise 1 – Breath Counting Meditation

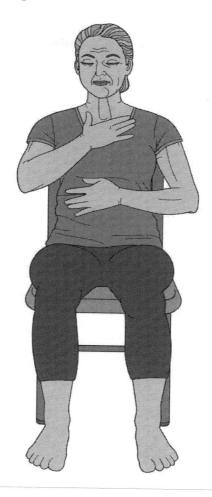

Step 1: Sit up tall on your chair in a stable position. Your legs should be hip-width apart, with your knees bent at a 90-degree angle stacked above your knees. Press your feet firmly against the floor and spread your toes as wide as possible.

Step 2: Squeeze your shoulder blades together to open the front of the chest. Lower your shoulders, and nod your chin slightly toward your chest to open the back of the neck. Relax your jaw.

Step 3: Place one hand just below your ribcage in the middle of your belly and the palm of your other hand on the center of your sternum or chest.

Step 4: Close your eyes. Focus on the sensation of the breath as it enters your nose and exits through your mouth. You may feel your heart beating under your palm and gentle expansion and contraction through the torso as you breathe. Connect with your body's subtle movements, sensations, and sounds.

Step 5: This is a breath-counting meditation. One breath is counted as an inhalation through the nose and an exhalation through the mouth. Start counting your breaths up to the number 10. If you notice your mind starts to stray, begin again at zero. It is much more challenging than it first seems. Sometimes you'll end up riding a train of thought for miles before you realize with a start, "Dang, I was supposed to be counting my breaths!"

Step 6: Once you've counted successfully to 10 breaths, start over and count to 15. Then start over and count to 20. After you count to 20, see how high you can go before a new thought arises. Once it does, start again at zero. Who knows, someday you could get to 100!

Exercise 2 – Full Body Relaxation

Step 1: Lie down on a firm mattress or sofa. Your legs should be hip-width apart. Use a thin pillow behind your head if you need support.

Step 2: Place one hand just below your ribcage in the middle of your belly and the palm of your other hand on the center of your sternum or chest.

Step 3: Close your eyes. Focus on the sensation of the breath as it enters your nose and exits through your mouth. You may feel your heart beating under your palm and gentle expansion and contraction through the torso as you breathe. Connect with your body's subtle movements, sensations, and sounds. Stay with your natural breath pace through this whole meditation.

Step 4: Once calm, position your arms alongside your body with your palms facing upward.

Step 5: Start the body scan at the top of the head, and in your mind's eye, relax it as you say to yourself, "I relax my scalp."

Step 6: Pause at least 1 to 3 complete breath cycles before moving on to the next body part.

Step 7: Repeat these steps as you relax each body part from head to toe:

- Forehead, eyes, cheeks, jaw, lips, mouth, and chin
- The tongue, the back of the throat, the heart, and the lungs
- The left shoulder, elbow, wrist, and tips of the fingers
- The chest
- The right shoulder, elbow, wrist, and tips of the fingers.
- The diaphragm
- The belly, the internal organs
- The left hip, knee, ankle, and tips of the toes
- The reproductive organs
- The right hip, knee, ankle, and tips of the toes

Step 8: Finish by saying to yourself, "I relax my whole body."

Step 9: Stay here as long as you wish, feeling the deep relaxation of your whole body. When ready to finish the meditation, you can wiggle your toes and fingers and stretch your body.

Exercise 3 – Mindfulness Meditation

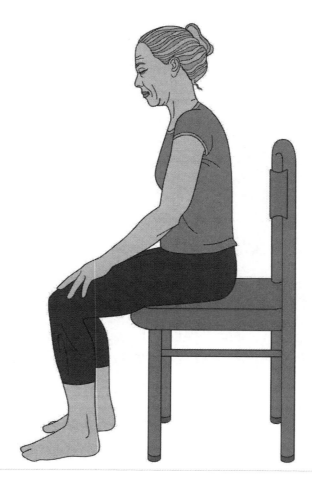

Step 1: Sit up tall on your chair.

Step 2: Place one hand just below your ribcage in the middle of your belly and the palm of your other hand on the center of your sternum or chest.

Step 3: Close your eyes. Focus on the sensation of the breath as it enters your nose and exits through your mouth. You may feel your heart beating under your palm and gentle expansion and contraction through the torso as you breathe. Connect with your body's subtle movements, sensations, and sounds. Stay with your innate breath pace through this whole meditation.

Step 4: When ready to begin, place your palms on your lap or in one of the mudras described above. Imagine that you see a river flowing before you. Visualize the river, the time of day, and the quality of the light.

Step 5: Observe your thoughts as they arrive. Once you notice that you have a thought, you can label it a "thought." Visualize placing your thoughts on a leaf in the river, and watch them float away.

Step 6: Return to your breath, and notice the pause between the inhalation and the exhalation.

Exercise 4 – Mantra Meditation

Step 1: Sit up tall on your chair.

Step 2: Place one hand just below your ribcage in the middle of your belly and the palm of your other hand on the center of your sternum or chest.

Step 3: Close your eyes. Focus on the sensation of the breath as it enters your nose and exits through your mouth. You may feel your heart beating under your palm and gentle expansion and contraction through the torso as you breathe. Connect with your body's subtle movements, sensations, and sounds. Stay with your innate breath pace through this whole meditation.

Step 4: When ready to begin, place your palms on your lap or in a mudra. Choose a word, phrase, mantra, or prayer with special personal meaning or resonance. It could be as simple as "love" or an affirmation such as "I am strong" or "I am kind." You can stay with this mantra as long as you feel comfortable. If you find your mind wandering, return to the breath, and repeat your mantra.

Exercise 5 – Loving Kindness Meditation

Step 1: Sit up tall on your chair.

Step 2: Place one hand just below your ribcage in the middle of your belly and the palm of your other hand on the center of your sternum or chest.

Step 3: Close your eyes. Focus on the sensation of the breath as it enters your nose and exits through your mouth. You may feel your heart beating under your palm and gentle expansion and contraction through the torso as you breathe. Connect with your body's subtle movements, sensations, and sounds. Stay with your innate breath pace through this whole meditation.

Step 4: When ready to begin, place your palms on your lap or in one of the mudras described previously. Imagine yourself in a state of complete and utter peace and harmony both in mind and body.

Step 5: Repeat three or four affirmations, such as:
- May I be happy
- May I be healthy
- May I be safe
- May I be loved

Step 6: Allow the essence of these affirmations to dissolve any doubt that you have the right to experience them. Give yourself time to connect with feelings of genuine warmth and self-compassion. Stay with this step of the meditation if it feels appropriate, or you can widen the circle.

Step 7: Think of someone who you deeply love and admire. Perhaps it's your parent, spouse, sibling, child, friend, or even the family pet. Visualize them, repeat the following affirmations, and send them this feeling of joy:
- May you be happy
- May you be healthy
- May you be safe
- May you be loved

Step 8: You can repeat the previous step with as many people (or animals) as you wish. More advanced practices include cultivating this feeling of joy, if it is sincere, and sending it to those you dislike.

Step 9: You can shift your loving kindness meditation to the collective. You can repeat the following affirmations and send this feeling of joy out into the world without conditions:
- May we all be happy
- May we all be healthy
- May we all be safe
- May we all be loved

Step 10: When you're ready, you can open your eyes. You can tap into the feelings of well-being generated during this meditation throughout the day by remembering your loving kindness practice and taking a few slow deep breaths.

Exercise 6 – Heart Chakra Meditation

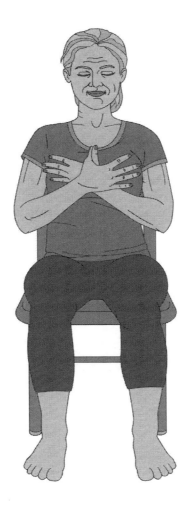

Step 1: Sit up tall on your chair.

Step 2: Place one hand just below your ribcage and the palm of your other hand on the center of your sternum or chest.

Step 3: Focus on the sensation of the breath as it enters your nose and exits through your mouth. You may feel your heart beating under your palm and gentle expansion and contraction through the torso as you breathe. Connect with your body's subtle movements, sensations, and sounds.

Step 4: To begin, rub the palms of your hands together until you feel them warming up. Once they are warm, turn your palms to face your body and then bring the pads of your thumbs together with your palms still facing the body to create garuda mudra, an eagle-shaped hand position.

Step 5: Place your hands over your chest, with your palms pressed against the sternum. Close your eyes. As you breathe, visualize that you are inhaling light into your heart. Connect with the beating of your heart as it pumps below your palms.

Step 6: Add the box breath. Inhale for four, hold for four, exhale for four, and hold the exhale for four. Notice how you become more aware of your heartbeat when you pause between your breaths. Include as many box breaths as you wish.

Step 7: Feel the warmth and light of your heart circulate through your body. Connect with this profound energy of love and include a mantra if it feels good for you, "I love myself."

CHAPTER 16 | A BRIEF HISTORY OF YOGA

Overview

Yoga is an ancient Indian spiritual practice with roots in the Indus Valley of present-day Pakistan. Archaeological evidence of yogic practices dating from before 2700 BC has been unearthed there. Yoga comes from Sanskrit and signifies the concept of yoking or uniting individual and universal consciousness, mind and body, human and nature. Individuals from any religious background can practice yoga.

Yogic traditions were passed down orally from guru to disciple until 200 BC when Maharishi Patanjali, a great sage and scribe, codified these teachings about Hatha yoga in the *Yoga Sutras*. The *Yoga Sutras* describe the eight limbs of yoga and provide a holistic lifestyle philosophy for yoga students. Hatha yoga is the foundation from which all other yoga styles later emerged.

The eight limbs of yoga include ethical standards, self-discipline, yoga asana (poses), pranayama, sensory transcendence, concentration, meditation, and the state of samadhi (ecstasy), which follows a dedicated practice of the abovementioned principles.

The first two limbs of yoga, ethical standards, and self-discipline, are sometimes overlooked in contemporary yoga practices. The current focus is on yoga asanas and, to a lesser degree, pranayama, and meditation. The yamas and niyamas offer ancient guidance for living a life of tranquility and peace that is still relevant and worth thoughtful consideration.

The Five Yamas (Ethical Standards)

Ahimsa (non-violence) – Ahimsa is the practice of peace. Violence can be physical, mental, or emotional harm toward the self and others. It is common to react with judgment, criticism, anger, or irritation on a daily basis when things don't go your way. Manifestations of violence include anything from the voice in your head that scolds you for making a mistake to the alarming rise of troll behavior on social media.

Violence is inherent in human nature; the goal is to live your life inflicting less violence on yourself and those around you. Ahimsa is an invitation to invite more compassion into your life. What does that look like? Once you notice and identify habitual adverse reactions towards yourself or others, you slowly replace them with kindness, acceptance, and love. At first, practicing compassion can be difficult and frustrating. But keep trying. Sooner rather than later, that practice will lead to perfection.

Satya (truthfulness) – Satya urges us to live and speak our truth. In honesty, we find an anchor to live a life of respect, honor, and integrity. Truth is also mindful of ahimsa, of non-violence, and makes it possible to negotiate difficult situations with respect for ourselves and others as we set boundaries. It also means ensuring that you treat others with the highest regard. Cultivate thoughts, words, and actions aligned with your truth and invite the energies into your life that encourage you to bloom into your highest self.

Asteya (non-stealing) – Asetya can be defined as refraining from taking what is not yours. Keep yourself and others from committing theft of mind, word, or action. At the societal level, asteya opposes social injustice, exploitation, and oppression.

Brahmacharya (continence) – Brahmacharya is the principle of controlling physical impulses and excess. Courage and strength are necessary to break the bonds that attach us to our excesses and addictions. Each time you overcome these impulses, you become stronger, healthier, and wiser.

Aparigraha (non-coveting) – Aparigraha urges you to release everything you do not need, possessing only as much as necessary. Take inventory of your possessions, don't let them own you! And if you have more than enough, consider this a call to cull and donate or redistribute these objects to those in need.

The Five Niyamas (Self-Discipline)

Shaucha (purification and cleanliness) – Shaucha is the first principle of Patanjali's five observances. Think of it as "do not pollute." Surround yourself with purity in all senses. Take in delicious and healthy food and drink. Feed your mind with nourishing and inspiring books, movies, and music. Engage in relationships with people who stimulate and support you. Ensure that your home is clean and in a state of harmony. When possible, try to use ecologically friendly forms of transportation such as walking or biking.

Samtosha (contentment) – Samtosha refers to finding satisfaction with what you have. Our society teaches us that material riches are the path to lasting happiness. Though material security is nothing to be scoffed at, it does not guarantee a joyous life. Get into the habit of naming three things you are grateful for first thing in the morning and again before you fall asleep.

Tapas (asceticism and self-discipline) – Tapas is defined as willpower. Doing the thing. Yes, that thing. The one you've been putting off that will positively affect your life. Tapas builds the self-discipline and personal strength necessary to become more focused, dedicated, and in tune with your goals. Harnessing your focus transforms unconscious impulses and poor behavior into intentional actions that will improve your life.

Svadhyaya (self-study and self-reflection) – Svadhyaya is the act of contemplating life's hard-earned lessons. Life gives us endless opportunities to learn more about ourselves and others during our time on Earth. Flaws, weaknesses, and mistakes can be composted into deep knowledge and growth. Self-examination can serve as a mirror to see your conscious and unconscious motives, thoughts, and desires more clearly. Sacred and spiritual texts and teachers can guide those called deeper into svadhyaya.

Ishvara Pranidhana (devotion and self-surrender) – Ishvara Pranidhana is the dedication of one's practice to a higher power. This intention infuses your yoga practice with grace, inner peace, and love. It is the fusion of the self with the divine.

These principles are an invitation to approach each day with greater consciousness. If any of these ethical standards or self-discipline concepts resonate with you, take the time to consider how you can integrate them into your daily life.

Types of Yoga

Over time, yoga branched in many directions as gurus interpreted, defined, and refined styles and disciplines. There are more than 11 styles, some of which are described below.

Hatha – Translated from Sanskrit ha (sun) and tha (moon), Hatha yoga harmonizes masculine and feminine energies within the body through practicing the eight limbs of yoga. The asanas are practiced slowly and held longer than other yoga styles. Hatha yoga is the genesis of all yoga styles developed in India and Pakistan.

Iyengar – Developed by B.K.S Iyengar in 1936, this style of yoga focuses on using blocks and straps to help students practice correct alignment and posture. It includes more than 200 yoga asanas and 14 different types of pranayama.

Ashtanga – K. Pattabhi Jois developed this form of yoga in the early 1900s. It includes a set of six specific routines of incremental difficulty levels and is incredibly dynamic and challenging. The asanas blend with flowing movements, also known as vinyasa.

Vinyasa – Unlike Ashtanga yoga, vinyasa does not comprise a set routine. The asanas merge through fluid movements and breath, yet the routine can vary from class to class. The guru T Krishnamacharya had a significant role in influencing how this style of yoga developed.

Kundalini – Kundalini yoga integrates chanting, singing, breath exercises, and repetitive movements to wake up the energy of spiritual awareness, or shakti, at the base of the spine. It was introduced to the West by Yogi Bhajan in the 1960s.

Hot Yoga – Hot yoga is based on the teachings of B. C. Ghoush and reached cult-like levels under the now-disgraced guru Bikram Choudhury during the 1970s. It consists of 26 postures done repeatedly during an hour-and-a-half class in a room heated up to 105 °F (41 °C).

Yin – Yin (stable, unmoving, receptive) is a Taoist principle, and this style of yoga originated in China and Tawain more than 2000 years ago. It consists of holding active stretches for two to seven minutes, supported by props to help deepen or ease the stretch to loosen up and relax the connective tissue. It focuses on opening up the lower body, especially the hips.

Restorative – Restorative yoga is similar to Yin yoga, except restorative yoga has no active stretch. Props support the body entirely, and practitioners hold stretches for extended periods to deeply relax the body.

Prenatal – Prenatal yoga is tailored to the rapidly changing needs of women throughout pregnancy. Prenatal yoga ensures that poses are safely modified so that women and their babies reap the benefits of the practice.

Chair – In 1979, a yoga teacher named Alice Christensen created a series of yoga poses that included postures in chairs. In 1982, Lakshmi Voelker began chair yoga after she saw that one of her students in her thirties, who had severe arthritis, couldn't complete specific floor exercises. Chair Yoga allows folks from all walks of life to practice yoga asana, pranayama, and meditation. They are skills to practice over a lifetime.

The Chakras

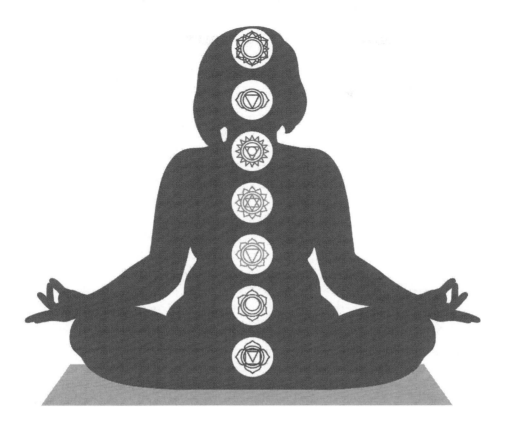

The chakras (wheels or disks) are an ancient concept first documented between 1500 and 1200 BC in the Vedas, four ancient scriptures which underpin the foundations of Hinduism. They can be considered energetic points that describe how energy flows through the human body. The spine has seven primary chakras along its length, but many lesser-known chakras exist throughout the body.

Each chakra corresponds to a specific region of the body, the function of nearby organs and nerves, and distinct emotional and spiritual states. The chakras are sometimes described as being "out of balance," meaning that the qualities specific to a particular chakra may be more or less present in an individual. It is possible to utilize different yoga asanas, pranayama, and even meditation to connect with the chakras so that energy circulates freely through the body.

Muladhara (root) chakra – Situated near the tailbone, the root chakra is symbolized by the color red and the element earth. It primarily deals with concerns related to survival, such as food and financial security. When out of balance, this chakra can manifest as anxiety about one's material stability, fear of the unknown, and an inability to focus. Physical symptoms include pain in the lower back, hips, prostate gland, and irregular menstrual cycles. Optimally, this chakra makes one feel more grounded, stable, and equipped with the strength to face life's continuous changes.

Svadhisthana (sacral) chakra – The sacral chakra is situated about three to four finger widths below the belly button. It is associated with sexual and creative energy and is symbolized by the color orange and the element of water. Individuals with sacral chakra imbalance might tend to overindulge in food, sex, or co-dependency in relationships to mask an underlying fear of abandonment. Physical symptoms include adrenal fatigue, digestive issues of the large intestine, and pain in the sacral area of the spine. When this chakra is in harmony, it shines a light on emotional interconnectivity, creativity, and innovation.

Manipura (solar plexus) chakra – This chakra can be found in the upper abdomen or stomach area. It is symbolized by the color yellow and the element of fire. It exemplifies the relationship to self. An imbalance of the solar plexus chakra can lead to a short temper, controlling behavior, and a lack of empathy for others. It can also reveal itself through insecurity, neediness, and passive-aggressiveness. Physical ailments can manifest in the liver, gallbladder, pancreas, stomach, and small intestine. At its best, this chakra radiates confidence, wisdom, and the capacity to show up authentically in the world.

Anahata (heart) chakra – The heart chakra, symbolized by the color green and the element of air, is located just above the heart. It unites the lower chakras related to materiality with the higher, more spiritual chakras. It focuses on the receptive and renewable nature of love, giving and receiving, and the formation of healthy relationships. Out of balance, this can look like putting the needs of others before oneself to the point of detriment, being taken advantage of, and challenges in setting one's boundaries. Conversely, it can look like shutting oneself off from love, armoring the heart, and reluctance to trust others. Physical symptoms include upper back and shoulder pain and circulatory and respiratory system issues. The heart chakra in tune emanates a deep sense of wholeness, expansiveness, and unconditional love.

Vishuddha (throat) chakra – Situated in the throat and symbolized by the color turquoise and the element of sound, this chakra relates to communication, expressing oneself honestly and clearly, and speaking from the heart. It delights in self-expression. When the throat chakra is out of equilibrium, it can be observed in those who constantly interrupt others, have difficulty listening, tell white lies, or otherwise obscure the truth. It can also be noticed in those who struggle to express their thoughts and opinions. Infirmity of the ears, mouth, lips, teeth, tongue, and thyroid gland can all manifest when this chakra is out of balance. The throat chakra is a conduit for spreading equanimity and truth when exalted.

Ajna (third eye) chakra – The color indigo and the element of light represent the third eye chakra. It is located in the center of the forehead, between the eyebrows. It sparks intuition and imagination, building trust in what is not always visible to the naked eye. Out of balance, this chakra can look like those who struggle to complete daily tasks, stay focused on their goals, or prefer to escape the material world through esoteric or spiritual practices. Conversely, they may feel completely disconnected from spirituality or belief in a higher power. Physical manifestations of imbalance include headaches, sinus infections, and general fatigue. The spiritual and material worlds align when the third eye chakra is in harmony.

Sahasrara (crown) chakra – Found at the top of the head, the crown chakra is symbolized by the color violet and the element of spirit. The seventh chakra is to be acknowledged, not balanced per se, as it is a portal to universal consciousness and represents nirvana, a state of enlightenment. The crown chakra is infinite and divine. It is possible to spend a lifetime investigating and integrating the energies of the six lower chakras on a quest for mental, physical, and spiritual balance.

CONCLUSION

Yoga with a chair is an empowering way to explore movement in a new context. Pain, illness, injuries, misfortune, surgery, the aging process; when these uninvited guests knock at the door, it can be challenging to say "Hello," "Welcome," or "What is the lesson here?" Resistance is a matter of course; your gut reaction might be to spray paint "GO AWAY!" and lock the door to emphasize your point. It's human nature to reject changes, especially those you haven't chosen yourself, which shift your life in an entirely unintended way.

I hope this book, *Chair Yoga for Seniors*, provides you with the tools to stand on the edge of that resistance and experiment with breathing into it, observing it, and expanding its boundaries. And that the diaphragmatic breath, meditation, and conscious movement connect you with your innate grace, courage, and wisdom. The benefits of these practices are limitless. Taking the time to reconnect with your body and its unique capacity to express itself through movement with self-acceptance and enthusiasm is invaluable.

I can consider this endeavor a success if you felt included and inspired to learn more about chair yoga. I aspired to make it easy for anyone who wants to learn more about these ancient practices to follow along. Advocating for accessible yoga is my passion. Thanks for joining me, fellow chair yoga practitioners!

Let's stay in touch!

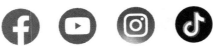

@dharmabumsyoga

PLEASE LEAVE A REVIEW!

If you enjoyed this book, please take 60 seconds to leave a review on Amazon! I'd love to hear your thoughts about Chair Yoga for Seniors. Did you find the poses easy to follow? Were the instructions clear and concise? Did you notice any flexibility or overall well-being improvements after practicing chair yoga? Your feedback is valuable and can help others decide if this book is right for them. Please leave a review and share your experience. Thank you so much!

Scan QR code:

REFERENCES

Abdominal muscles: Anatomy and function. Cleveland Clinic. (n.d.). Retrieved August 8, 2022, from https://my.clevelandclinic.org/health/body/21755-abdominal-muscles

Anne Asher, C. P. T. (2022, March 4). What does your latissimus Dorsi do? Verywell Health. Retrieved August 7, 2022, from https://www.verywellhealth.com/latissimus-dorsi-muscle-anatomy-297067

Arch, L. (2021, June 1). 10 poses to avoid if you're pregnant: Wellness: Myfitnesspal. MyFitnessPal Blog. Retrieved September 4, 2022, from References https://blog.myfitnesspal.com/10-poses-avoid-youre-pregnant/

Ballestrini, C. (2017, August 11). Rotator cuff tear: Orthopedics & sports medicine. UConn Health. Retrieved August 5, 2022, from https://health.uconn.edu/orthopedics-sports-medicine/conditions-and-treatments/where-does-it-hurt/shoulder/rotator-cuff-tear/#:~:text=Rotator%20cuff%20tears%20as%20a,%2C%20 lacrosse%2C%20and%20ice%20hockey.

Basavaraddi, D. I. V. (n.d.). Yoga: Its origin, history and development - yogamdniy.nic. in. Retrieved August 20, 2022, from http://yogamdniy.nic.in/WriteReadData/LINKS/ File577a4a83f0b-996b-4119-842d-60790971e651.pdf

Bheekoo-Shah, F. (2022, April 24). 5 meditation practices in Islam. About Islam. Retrieved March 2, 2023, from https://aboutislam.net/family-life/self-development/5-meditation-practices-in-islam/

Bhavanani , Y. M. D. (n.d.). Yoga Sutras of Patanjali: An overview - ICYER. Retrieved August 20, 2022, from http://icyer.com/documents/patanjali.pdf

Boynton, E. (2021, January 27). What happens in the brain during meditation? Right as Rain by UW Medicine. Retrieved March 1, 2023, from https://rightasrain.uwmedicine.org/mind/well-being/science-behind-meditation#:~:text=Through%20meditation%2C%20you%20are%20essentially,%2C%20depression%2C%20stress%20 and%20anxiety.

Brennan, MD , D. (n.d.). Proprioception: What it is, disorder, symptoms, and more. WebMD. Retrieved August 4, 2022, from https://www.webmd.com/brain/what-is-proprioception

Bulletin 235: Office ergonomics - arm, hand and wrist hazards. SAFE Work Manitoba. (n.d.). Retrieved August 12, 2022, from https://www.safemanitoba.com/Resources/Pages/bulletin-235.aspx

Burgin, T. (2020, November 28). The five niyamas of yoga: Definition & practice tips. Yoga Basics. Retrieved January 5, 2023, from https://www.yogabasics.com/learn/the-five-niyamas-of-yoga/

Burgin, T. (2021, March 29). The five yamas of yoga: Definition & practice tips. Yoga Basics. Retrieved January 5, 2023, from https://www.yogabasics.com/learn/the-five-yamas-of-yoga/

Cameron, Y. (2023, March 15). Everything you've ever wanted to know about the 7 chakras in the body. mindbodygreen. https://www.mindbodygreen.com/articles/7-chakras-for-beginners

Chair yoga for seniors: Reduce pain and improve health. DailyCaring. (2021, March 16). Retrieved August 20, 2022, from https://dailycaring.com/chair-yoga-for-seniors-reduce-pain-and-improve-health-video/#:~:text=The%20benefits%20of%20chair%20yoga,and%20builds%20strength%20and%20balance.

Chair yoga poses: How to get started with chair yoga. Chair Yoga Poses | How to get started with chair yoga. (n.d.). Retrieved August 20, 2022, from https://www.uaex.uada.edu/life-skills-wellness/health/physical-activity-resources/chair-yoga.aspx

Common hip injuries. Weiss Memorial Hospital. (2022, January 24). Retrieved August 9, 2022, from https://www.weisshospital.com/our-services/orthopedics/hip-care/common-hip-injuries/

Common neck injuries and conditions. Common Neck Conditions Symptoms & Causes | Dignity Health. (n.d.). Retrieved March 9, 2023, from https://www.dignityhealth.org/conditions-and-treatments/orthopedics/common-neck-injuries-and-conditions

Cronkleton, E. (2019, December 17). How to stretch tight hips: 12 stretches and instructions. Healthline. Retrieved August 9, 2022, from https://www.healthline.com/health/exercise-fitness/how-to-stretch-hips#hip-flexor-stretches

REFERENCES

Curtis, L., & Ammerman, MD , J. M. (2022, January 4). *Cervical spine anatomy (neck) - spineuniverse.* Retrieved March 9, 2023, from https://www.spineuniverse.com/anatomy/cervical-spine-anatomy-neck

Davis, A. (2020, December 20). *Chair yoga for pregnancy. Bliss Baby Yoga.* Retrieved August 20, 2022, from https://www.blissbabyyoga.com/chair-yoga-for-pregnancy/#:~:text=There%20are%20so%20many%20benefits,do%20with%20ease%20are%20limited.

Deslippe, P. (2019, June 20). *Yoga landed in the U.S. way earlier than you'd think-and fitness was not the point. History.com.* Retrieved September 3, 2022, from https://www.history.com/news/yoga-vivekananda-america

Disabled World. (2022, April 14). *Seniors and disability yoga exercises and information. Disabled World.* Retrieved August 20, 2022, from https://www.disabled-world.com/fitness/exercise/yoga/

Dunleavy, B. P., Rodriguez, D., Tanenbaum, S., Vann, M. R., Scott, J. A., By, & McCoy, K. (n.d.). *10 common foot problems and how to manage them. EverydayHealth.com.* Retrieved August 10, 2022, from https://www.everydayhealth.com/foot-health-pictures/common-foot-problems.aspx#:~:text=And%20many%20foot%20problems%2C%20including,sign%20of%20a%20systemic%20problem.

Encyclopædia Britannica, inc. (n.d.). *Latissimus dorsi. Encyclopædia Britannica.* Retrieved August 7, 2022, from https://www.britannica.com/science/latissimus-dorsi

Gasnick PT, DPT, K. (2021, November 15). *Arm muscle anatomy and function. Verywell Health.* Retrieved March 9, 2023, from https://www.verywellhealth.com/arm-muscle-anatomy-5180227#:~:text=There%20are%2024%20different%20muscles,(back%20of%20the%20arm).

Gerritsen, R. J. S., & Band, G. P. H. (2018, October 9). *Breath of life: The respiratory vagal stimulation model of contemplative activity. Frontiers in human neuroscience.* Retrieved April 13, 2023, from https://www.ncbi.nlm.nih.gov/pmc/articles/PMC6189422/

Get to know the Seven chakras. *Yoloha Yoga.* (n.d.). https://yolohayoga.com/blogs/yoloha-life/get-to-know-the-seven-chakras

REFERENCES

Glass MD, D. (2019, January 30). *Demystifying pelvic organ prolapse. UChicago Medicine.* https://www.uchicagomedicine.org/forefront/womens-health-articles/de-mystifying-pelvic-organ-prolapses#:~:text=It%20is%20very%20common%2C%20with,for%20it%20in%20their%20lifetime.

Government of Canada, C. C. for O. H. and S. (2022, December 4). *Working in a sitting position - overview : Osh answers. Canadian Centre for Occupational Health and Safety.* Retrieved December 4, 2022, from https://www.ccohs.ca/oshanswers/ergonomics/sitting/sitting_overview.html

Gupta, A., Gupta, R., Sood, S., & Arkham, M. (2014, February). *Pranayam for treatment of chronic obstructive pulmonary disease: Results from a randomized, controlled trial. Integrative medicine (Encinitas, Calif.).* Retrieved October 24, 2022, from https://www.ncbi.nlm.nih.gov/pmc/articles/PMC4684118/

Harika, Elizabeth, Mary, Cremets, N., Conaty, A., Viswanathan, A. S., Rao, D., Kannan, S., Koers, L., Relo, Mandelia, K., boro, M., Sander, J., Goldman, M., O'Connor, T., & Blanc, C. (2023, March 2). *Ashtanga yoga: Definition, principles, practices & history. Yoga Basics.* Retrieved April 25, 2023, from https://www.yogabasics.com/learn/ashtanga-yoga/

Hip anatomy. Physiopedia. (n.d.). Retrieved August 9, 2022, from https://www.physio-pedia.com/Hip_Anatomy

Hip injury prevention tips. Timothy J. Jackson, M.D.- Hip Arthroscopic & Hip Replacement Surgery. (n.d.). Retrieved August 9, 2022, from https://www.timothyjacksonmd.com/blog/hip-injury-prevention-tips-24483/

Hoffman, M. (n.d.). *Knee (human anatomy): Function, parts, conditions, treatments. WebMD.* Retrieved August 10, 2022, from https://www.webmd.com/pain-management/knee-pain/picture-of-the-knee

Hoth, H. W. P. S. (2020, September 30). *7 types of hand injuries you should know about. Houston Wrist Pain Specialists: Elbow, Hand & Finger Surgery | HSST.* Retrieved August 6, 2022, from https://carpaltunnelpros.com/2019/12/17/types-of-hand-injuries/

REFERENCES

Howard, A. (2022, April 19). *Meditation can change your brain waves: Here's how.* Psych Central. Retrieved March 2, 2023, from https://psychcentral.com/health/meditation-brain-waves#what-happens-in-the-brain

Inverarity, DO, L. (2021, November 14). *The 4 muscles that make up the rotator cuff.* Verywell Health. Retrieved August 5, 2022, from https://www.verywellhealth.com/the-rotator-cuff-2696385#:~:text=The%20acronym%20SITS%20is%20often,%2C%20teres%20minor%2C%20and%20subscapularis.

John Peloza, M. D. (n.d.). *Causes of lower back pain.* Spine. Retrieved August 7, 2022, from https://www.spine-health.com/conditions/lower-back-pain/causes-lower-back-pain

Kamani, J. (2010, February 15). *Hip flexor tightness linked to chronic injuries in student-athlete runners: Trackmedic: National Scholastic Athletics Foundation.* National Scholastic Sports Foundation. Retrieved August 9, 2022, from https://www.nationalscholastic.org/trackmedic/article/hip_flexor_tightness_linked_to_chronic_injuries_in_student_athlete_runners

Know your brain: Vestibular system. @neurochallenged. (n.d.). Retrieved August 4, 2022, from https://neuroscientificallychallenged.com/posts/know-your-brain-vestibular-system#:~:text=The%20vestibular%20system%20is%20a,during%20movement%2C%20and%20maintain%20posture.

Kurre, A., Straumann, D., van Gool, C. J., Gloor-Juzi, T., & Bastiaenen, C. H. (2012, March 22). *Gender differences in patients with dizziness and unsteadiness regarding self-perceived disability, anxiety, depression, and its associations.* BMC ear, nose, and throat disorders. Retrieved August 4, 2022, from https://www.ncbi.nlm.nih.gov/pmc/articles/PMC3352112/#:~:text=found%20that%2012.7%25%20of%20women,of%20experienced%20handicap%20%5B4%5D.

Larsen, K. (2021, February 10). *Vestibular Impairment and its association to the neck and TMJ.* MSK Neurology. Retrieved August 4, 2022, from https://mskneurology.com/vestibular-impairment-and-its-association-to-the-neck-and-tmj/

Lau, C., Yu, R., & Woo, J. (2015). *Effects of a 12-week Hatha yoga intervention on cardiorespiratory endurance, muscular strength and endurance, and flexibility in Hong Kong Chinese adults: A controlled clinical trial.* Evidence-based complementary *and alternative medicine : eCAM. Retrieved August 6, 2022, from https://www.ncbi.nlm.nih.gov/pmc/articles/PMC4475706/*

Lockard, T. (2022, February 2). How volunteering improves mental health. NAMI. Retrieved December 4, 2022, from https://www.nami.org/Blogs/NAMI-Blog/February-2022/How-Volunteering-Improves-Mental-Health#:~:text=A%202020%20study%20conducted%20in,those%20who%20did%20not%20volunteer.

Lothian, J. A. (2011). Lamaze breathing: What every pregnant woman needs to know. The Journal of perinatal education. Retrieved March 8, 2023, from https://www.ncbi.nlm.nih.gov/pmc/articles/PMC3209750/

Lung Disease. Pennmedicine.org. (n.d.). Retrieved October 24, 2022, from https://www.pennmedicine.org/for-patients-and-visitors/patient-information/conditions-treated-a-to-z/lung-disease

Ma, X., Yue, Z.-Q., Gong, Z.-Q., Zhang, H., Duan, N.-Y., Shi, Y.-T., Wei, G.-X., & Li, Y.-F. (2017, June 6). The effect of diaphragmatic breathing on attention, negative affect and stress in healthy adults. Frontiers in psychology. Retrieved August 13, 2022, from https://www.ncbi.nlm.nih.gov/pmc/articles/PMC5455070/#:~:text=Psychological%20studies%20have%20revealed%20breathing,et%20al.%2C%202015).

Ma, Y.-tao. (2011). Piriformis muscle. Piriformis Muscle - an overview | ScienceDirect Topics. Retrieved August 9, 2022, from https://www.sciencedirect.com/topics/neuroscience/piriformis-muscle#:~:text=The%20piriformis%20muscle%20originates%20at,the%20femur%20in%20the%20acetabulum.

Mayo Foundation for Medical Education and Research. (2022, April 29). A beginner's guide to meditation. Mayo Clinic. Retrieved August 13, 2022, from https://www.mayoclinic.org/tests-procedures/meditation/in-depth/meditation/art-20045858

Mayo Foundation for Medical Education and Research. (2020, August 18). Benign paroxysmal positional vertigo (BPPV). Mayo Clinic. Retrieved August 4, 2022, from https://www.mayoclinic.org/diseases-conditions/vertigo/symptoms-causes/syc-20370055

Mayo Foundation for Medical Education and Research. (2022, December 6). How to squeeze in Kegels All Day long. Mayo Clinic. https://www.mayoclinic.org/healthy-lifestyle/womens-health/in-depth/kegel-exercises/art-20045283

REFERENCES

Mayo Foundation for Medical Education and Research. (2021, May 11). Knee pain. Mayo Clinic. Retrieved August 10, 2022, from https://www.mayoclinic.org/diseases-conditions/knee-pain/symptoms-causes/syc-20350849

Mayo Foundation for Medical Education and Research. (2020, December 2). Meniere's disease. Mayo Clinic. Retrieved August 4, 2022, from https://www.mayoclinic.org/diseases-conditions/menieres-disease/symptoms-causes/syc-20374910

Mayo Foundation for Medical Education and Research. (2020, August 29). Why your core muscles matter. Mayo Clinic. Retrieved August 8, 2022, from https://www.mayoclinic.org/healthy-lifestyle/fitness/in-depth/core-exercises/art-20044751#:~:-text=Strong%20core%20muscles%20are%20also,also%20help%20improve%20back%20pain.

Mental health disorder statistics. Mental Health Disorder Statistics | Johns Hopkins Medicine. (2019, November 19). Retrieved November 14, 2022, from https://www.hopkinsmedicine.org/health/wellness-and-prevention/mental-health-disorder-statistics

Mental health. CMHA Ontario. (n.d.). Retrieved November 14, 2022, from https://ontario.cmha.ca/documents/connection-between-mental-and-physical-health/#:~:-text=The%20associations%20between%20mental%20and,of%20developing%20poor%20mental%20health.

Middle back pain. Middle Back Pain Symptoms & Causes | Dignity Health. (n.d.). Retrieved August 7, 2022, from https://www.dignityhealth.org/conditions-and-treatments/orthopedics/common-back-and-spine-injuries-and-conditions/middle-back-pain

Normal hand anatomy. Normal Hand Anatomy Colorado | Hand and Wrist Bones Lone Tree. (n.d.). Retrieved March 9, 2023, from https://www.orthotree.com/normal-hand-anatomy.html#:~:text=The%20hand's%20complex%20anatomy%20consists,that%20can%20affect%20our%20hands.

NHS. (n.d.). NHS choices. https://www.nhs.uk/conditions/pelvic-organ-prolapse/

Nunez, K. (2020, July 16). Kundalini yoga: Poses, benefits, steps for Beginners. Healthline. Retrieved April 25, 2023, from https://www.healthline.com/health/kundalini-yoga#about-kundalini-yoga

REFERENCES

Pilar. (2021, May 27). Anjali mudra meaning: The benefits of "Prayer hands" in yoga. Bodhi Surf + Yoga. Retrieved March 16, 2023, from https://www.bodhisurfyoga.com/meaning-of-anjali-mudra

Pranayama for self-soothing: 3 yogic breathing practices to cultivate peace. Kripalu. (2020, October 29). Retrieved August 13, 2022, from https://kripalu.org/resources/pranayama-self-soothing-3-yogic-breathing-practices-cultivate-peace?gclid=Cj0KC-Qjw54iXBhCXARIsADWpsG-if2gEIhkIr0E-k9TD3LWsuRZnIt6nwXIePCze1dbCBRS-XRkzC4SwaAqybEALw_wcB

Quinn, E. (2022, August 3). Anatomy and common injuries of the feet or ankles. Verywell Health. Retrieved August 10, 2022, from https://www.verywellhealth.com/foot-anatomy-and-physiology-3119204

Radley, D. C., Williams , R. D., Gunia, M. Z., Baumgartner, J. C., & Gumas, E. D. (2022, August 11). Americans, no matter the state they live in, die younger than people in many other countries. Commonwealth Fund. Retrieved November 14, 2022, from https://www.commonwealthfund.org/blog/2022/americans-no-matter-state-they-live-die-younger-people-many-other-countries

Rajah, U. S. (2022, July 18). Dhyana mudra (gesture of meditation): How to do, benefits. Fitsri. Retrieved March 16, 2023, from https://www.fitsri.com/yoga-mudras/dhyana-mudra#:~:text=Dhyana%20Mudra%20is%20a%20popular,joining%20both%20thumbs%20tips%20diagonally.

The real-world benefits of strengthening your core. Harvard Health. (2012, January 24). Retrieved August 8, 2022, from https://www.health.harvard.edu/healthbeat/the-real-world-benefits-of-strengthening-your-core#:~:text=Housework%2C%20fix-%2Dit%20work%2C,Balance%20and%20stability.

Rhomboids. Physiopedia. (n.d.). Retrieved August 7, 2022, from https://www.physio-pedia.com/Rhomboids

Riopel MSc., L. (2023, February 22). 28 best meditation techniques for beginners to learn. PositivePsychology.com. Retrieved March 1, 2023, from https://positivepsychology.com/meditation-techniques-beginners/

REFERENCES

Ross, A. (2016, March 9). Meditation history: Religious practice to mainstream trend. Time. Retrieved March 1, 2023, from https://time.com/4246928/meditation-history-buddhism/

Rotator cuff: Anatomy, common injuries & faqs. Cleveland Clinic. (n.d.). Retrieved August 5, 2022, from https://my.clevelandclinic.org/health/articles/21504-rotator-cuff#:~:text=The%20rotator%20cuff%20contains%20four,that%20helps%20rotate%20your%20arm.

Saxena, T., & Saxena, M. (2009, January). The effect of various breathing exercises (pranayama) in patients with bronchial asthma of mild to moderate severity. International journal of yoga. Retrieved October 24, 2022, from https://www.ncbi.nlm.nih.gov/pmc/articles/PMC3017963/

Scott, C. (2021, October 18). Repetitive strain injury. Repetitive Strain Injury: How to prevent, identify, and manage RSI. Retrieved August 12, 2022, from https://web.eecs.umich.edu/~cscott/rsi.html

Seladi-Schulman, J. (2018, August 27). Vagus nerve: Function, stimulation, and more. Healthline. Retrieved April 13, 2023, from https://www.healthline.com/human-body-maps/vagus-nerve#What-is-the-vagus-nerve?

Sharma, A., Madaan, V., & Petty, F. D. (2006). Exercise for mental health. Primary care companion to the Journal of clinical psychiatry. Retrieved November 14, 2022, from https://www.ncbi.nlm.nih.gov/pmc/articles/PMC1470658/

Smith, MD, D. G. (2006, November). Notes from the medical director grasping the importance of our hands. Retrieved August 7, 2022, from https://orthop.washington.edu/sites/default/files/files/16-6-document.pdf

Staff. (2020, September 17). Taking Vitamin D Twice a Day May Keep Vertigo Away. U.S. Pharmacist – The Leading Journal in Pharmacy. Retrieved August 4, 2022, from https://www.uspharmacist.com/article/taking-vitamin-d-twice-a-day-may-keep-vertigo-away#:~:text=Research%20published%20August%202020%20in,and%20sometimes%20dangerous%20physiologic%20symptom.

Strength and resistance training exercise. www.heart.org. (2020, July 18). Retrieved August 6, 2022, from https://www.heart.org/en/healthy-living/fitness/fitness-basics/strength-and-resistance-training-exercise#.VzDX8hUrLX8

REFERENCES

Sussex Publishers. (n.d.). An overview of meditation: Its origins and traditions. Psychology Today. Retrieved March 1, 2023, from https://www.psychologytoday.com/us/blog/meditation-modern-life/201307/overview-meditation-its-origins-and-traditions

Talasz, H., Kremser, C., Talasz, H. J., Kofler, M., & Rudisch, A. (2022, June 2). Breathing, (s)training and the pelvic floor-a basic concept. Healthcare (Basel, Switzerland). https://www.ncbi.nlm.nih.gov/pmc/articles/PMC9222935/

The difference between Yin and restorative yoga. YogaRenew. (2023, February 7). Retrieved April 25, 2023, from https://www.yogarenewteachertraining.com/the-difference-between-yin-and-restorative-yoga/#:~:text=In%20yin%20yoga%20the%20focus,deepen%20or%20ease%20the%20stretch.

The yoga sutras of patanjali - integral yoga studio. (n.d.). Retrieved August 20, 2022, from http://www.integralyogastudio.com/ysp/ysp-alex-bailey-long.pdf

U.S. Department of Health and Human Services. (n.d.). Anxiety disorders. National Institute of Mental Health. Retrieved November 14, 2022, from https://www.nimh.nih.gov/health/topics/anxiety-disorders

U.S. Department of Health and Human Services. (2018, March 6). Balance disorders. National Institute of Deafness and Other Communication Disorders. Retrieved August 4, 2022, from https://www.nidcd.nih.gov/health/balance-disorders#:~:text=About%2015%20percent%20of%20American,cause%20psychological%20and%20emotional%20hardship.

U.S. Department of Health and Human Services. (n.d.). Balance problems and disorders. National Institute on Aging. Retrieved August 4, 2022, from https://www.nia.nih.gov/health/balance-problems-and-disorders

U.S. Department of Health and Human Services. (n.d.). Meditation and mindfulness: What you need to know. National Center for Complementary and Integrative Health. Retrieved March 1, 2023, from https://www.nccih.nih.gov/health/meditation-and-mindfulness-what-you-need-to-know

U.S. National Library of Medicine. (n.d.). Arm injuries | arm disorders. MedlinePlus. Retrieved August 6, 2022, from https://medlineplus.gov/arminjuriesanddisorders.html

REFERENCES

Vagus nerve. Physiopedia. (n.d.). Retrieved February 14, 2023, from https://www. physio-pedia.com/Vagus_Nerve#:~:text=The%20vagus%20nerve%20runs%20 from,skull%20through%20the%20jugular%20foramen.

Vestibular rehabilitation exercises. Brain & Spine Foundation. (n.d.). Retrieved August 4, 2022, from https://www.brainandspine.org.uk/our-publications/our-fact-sheets/vestibular-rehabilitation-exercises/

WebMD. (n.d.). Common vitamins and supplements to treat vertigo. WebMD. Retrieved August 4, 2022, from https://www.webmd.com/vitamins/condition-1648/vertigo

What are brainwaves?: Brainworks Neurotherapy London. Brainworks Neurofeedback | The UK's Neurofeedback leaders since 2007. London clinic, home training and industry software developers. (2023, February 21). Retrieved March 3, 2023, from https://brainworksneurotherapy.com/about/faq/what-are-brainwaves/

What are the advantages of nose breathing vs. mouth breathing? Dental Logic. (2021, March 20). Retrieved March 8, 2023, from https://www.dentallogictruro.co.uk/what-are-the-advantages-of-nose-breathing-vs-mouth-breathing/

What happens in the brain during meditation? Right as Rain by UW Medicine. (2021, January 27). Retrieved August 13, 2022, from https://rightasrain.uwmedicine. org/mind/well-being/science-behind-meditation#:~:text=Meditation%20calms%20 down%20your%20sympathetic%20nervous%20system&text=Through%20meditation%2C%20you%20are%20essentially,%2C%20depression%2C%20stress%20 and%20anxiety.

What is Gyan Mudra? - definition from Yogapedia. Yogapedia.com. (n.d.). Retrieved March 16, 2023, from https://www.yogapedia.com/definition/6444/gyan-mudra#:~:-text=Definition%20%2D%20What%20does%20Gyan%20Mudra,Hindu%20and%20 Yoga%20traditions%20alike.

What is Hatha Yoga? - definition from Yogapedia. Yogapedia.com. (n.d.). Retrieved April 25, 2023, from https://www.yogapedia.com/definition/4977/hatha-yoga

What is Iyengar Yoga? - definition from Yogapedia. Yogapedia.com. (n.d.). Retrieved April 25, 2023, from https://www.yogapedia.com/definition/5017/iyengar-yoga

REFERENCES

What to do about rotator cuff tendinitis. Harvard Health. (2021, October 19). Retrieved August 5, 2022, from https://www.health.harvard.edu/pain/what-to-do-about-rotator-cuff-tendinitis#:~:text=The%20most%20common%20cause%20of%20shoulder%20pain%20is%20rotator%20cuff,arm%20up%20to%20the%20side.

Wikimedia Foundation. (2022, August 3). Accessible yoga. Wikipedia. Retrieved August 20, 2022, from https://en.wikipedia.org/wiki/Accessible_yoga#:~:text=Lakshmi%20Voelker%20(given%20her%20first,floor%20poses%20because%20of%20 arthritis.

Wikimedia Foundation. (2023, April 17). Bikram yoga. Wikipedia. Retrieved April 25, 2023, from https://en.wikipedia.org/wiki/Bikram_Yoga

Wikimedia Foundation. (2022, August 16). History of Christian meditation. Wikipedia. Retrieved March 2, 2023, from https://en.wikipedia.org/wiki/History_of_Christian_meditation

Wikimedia Foundation. (2022, October 24). Jewish meditation. Wikipedia. Retrieved March 2, 2023, from https://en.wikipedia.org/wiki/Jewish_meditation#:~:text=Jewish%20meditation%20includes%20practices%20of,philosophical%2C%20ethical%20or%20mystical%20ideas.

Wikimedia Foundation. (2023, May 8). Vedas. Wikipedia. https://en.wikipedia.org/wiki/Vedas

Wolf, A. (2022, June 21). Natural supplements for vestibular disorders. VeDA. Retrieved August 4, 2022, from https://vestibular.org/article/diagnosis-treatment/treatments/complementary-alternative-medicine/supplements/#:~:text=Neuritis%20%26%20Meniere%27s%20Disease-,L%2Dlysine,for%20reducing%20tinnitus%20and%20vertigo.

World Health Organization. (n.d.). Covid-19 pandemic triggers 25% increase in prevalence of anxiety and depression worldwide. World Health Organization. Retrieved November 14, 2022, from https://www.who.int/news/item/02-03-2022-covid-19-pandemic-triggers-25-increase-in-prevalence-of-anxiety-and-depression-worldwide

REFERENCES

World Health Organization. (n.d.). The Global Status Report on physical activity 2022. World Health Organization. Retrieved November 14, 2022, from https://www.who.int/teams/health-promotion/physical-activity/global-status-report-on-physical-activity-2022

Yin Yoga. Ekhart Yoga. (2022, May 26). Retrieved April 25, 2023, from https://www.ekhartyoga.com/resources/styles/yin-yoga#:~:text=Yin%20yoga%20is%20a%20quiet%20contemplative%20practice.&text=It%20targets%20the%20deepest%20tissues,yoga%20which%20targets%20the%20muscles.

Zaccaro, A., Piarulli, A., Laurino, M., Garbella, E., Menicucci, D., Neri, B., & Gemignani, A. (2018, September 7). How breath-control can change your life: A systematic review on psycho-physiological correlates of slow breathing. Frontiers in human neuroscience. Retrieved August 13, 2022, from https://www.ncbi.nlm.nih.gov/pmc/articles/PMC6137615/

FURTHER READING

Brach, T. (2004). *Radical acceptance: Embracing your life with the heart of a buddha.* Bantam Books.

Brown, C. B. (2007). *I thought it was just me (but it isn't): Women reclaiming power and courage in a culture of shame.* Gotham.

Chödrön, P. (2017). *When things fall apart: Heart advice for difficult times.* Thorsons Classics.

Chödrön, P. (2018). *The places that scare you: A guide to fearlessness in difficult times.* Shambhala.

Lad, V. (2006). *The Complete Book of Ayurvedic* Home Remedies. Piatkus.

Nestor, J. (2021). *Breath: The new science of a lost art.* Penguin Life.

Tiwari, M. (2016). *Women's power to heal: Through inner medicine.* Mother Om Media.

Printed in Great Britain
by Amazon

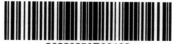

36220250R00108